CURE

DIABETES

NATURALLY

CURE

DIABETES

NATURALLY

A USERS GUIDE TO CURING TYPE 2 DIABETES WITHOUT DRUGS

JONATHAN PRINS

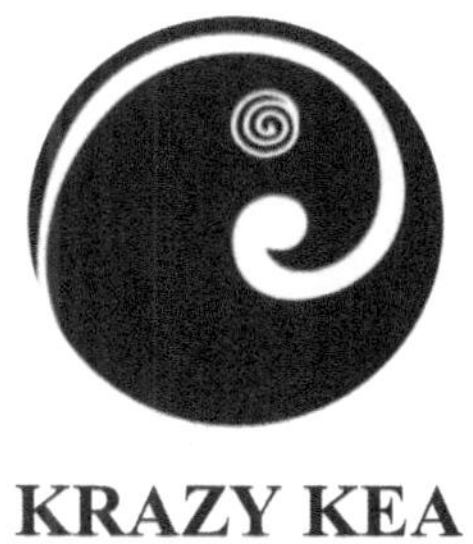

KRAZY KEA

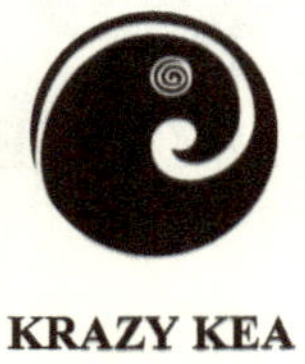

KRAZY KEA

To Freya,

We love you and miss you.

"Natural forces within us are the true healers of disease"
-Hippocrates

"Modern medicine is a negation of health. It isn't organized to serve human health, but only itself, as an institution. It makes more people sick than it heals"

-Ivan Illich

"The first wealth is health"
-Ralph Waldo Emerson

"It is reasonable to expect the doctor to recognize that science may not have all the answers to problems of health and healing"
-Norman Cousins

NOTICE TO READERS

This book was written with the intention of sharing information gathered from personal experience and from research done by nutritionists, scientists, doctors, healthcare professionals and many others.

The information contained in this book is intended for informational and educational purposes only, and should not be regarded as medical advice. Use discretion and consult your doctor or healthcare provider before you attempt anything recommended in this book.

The author, printer and publisher shall have no liability or responsibility to any person or entity with regards to any loss, damage, or injury caused or alleged to be caused either directly or indirectly by the information contained in this book.

The information contained in this book is not intended to diagnose or prescribe any form of treatment for any illness or medical condition. It is not to be used as a substitute for expert medical advice. Always consult with your doctor or healthcare provider before you begin a new regime or consider taking a new supplement.

Your doctor, naturopath or healthcare provider will also be able to recommend an exercise regime, nutritional supplements and dietary requirements that suit your particular profile as each individual situation is unique.

ACKNOWLEDGEMENTS

I wish to thank Mimi Kirk, Tim Ferriss, Professor Robert H. Lustig, Professor Roy Taylor, Dr. Stefan Ripich, Jim Healthy, Sean Croxton, Dr. Joel Fuhrman, Dr. Gabriel Cousens, Dr. Hans Michael Dosch, Dr. Michael Salter, Professor Len Harrison, Professor Peter Colman, Dr. Spiros Fourlanos, Dr. Fedon Lindberg, Dr. Neal Barnard, Patrick Holford and DeWayne McCulley firstly for doing the research and secondly for kindly giving me permission to use their names and works as references.

The way we view diseases and the way in which we treat those diseases is changing. These are some of the people who are showing us how to do this.

"Do not go where the path may lead; go instead where there is no path and leave a trail."

– Ralph Waldo Emerson

Table of Contents

This book was written to address issues of concern for people suffering from Type 2 Diabetes (AKA Adult Onset Diabetes) and similar metabolic illnesses such as Metabolic Syndrome, Metabolic Syndrome X, Cardiometabolic Syndrome, IRS (Insulin Resistance Syndrome), Reaven's Syndrome (after Gerald Reaven), CHAOS (in Australia) and Prediabetes.

TYPE 1 DIABETES: is an autoimmune disease which is a very different disease to type 2 diabetes. The recommendations in this book may be of benefit to people with type 1diabetes but is in no way intended to treat or cure it. Dr. Gabriel Cousens' raw vegan program for curing diabetes claims to have achieved dramatic results for type 1 diabetics too.

Type 1 diabetes is caused by damage done to the insulin producing cells of the pancreas. The body's own immune system attacks the pancreas' insulin producing cells hence the term autoimmune disease.

A study done in 1992 at The Hospital for Sick Children in Toronto, Canada, implicates cow's milk as a causative agent for type 1 diabetes. **Bovine serum albumin (BSA) a** milk protein contains the **ABBOS** epitope (**17-Amino-Acid Bovine Serum Albumin Peptide**) an albumin peptide containing 17 amino acids. The pancreatic beta-cell surface protein **P69** is an exact match for the ABBOS peptide. An infant's immune system cannot distinguish between the P69 protein and the ABBOS protein.

Antibodies that attack the ABBOS peptide now also selectively target, attack and destroy the insulin producing pancreatic beta-cells, which causes insulin-dependent type 1diabetes. While there are similarities between type 1 and type 2, they are different in terms of how they are acquired and how they progress inside the body.

This immune system's over-reaction to a milk protein seems to be something that only affects infants who do not yet have strong immune systems. There does not seem to be any risk to adults or adolescents. This is not the only cause for type 1 diabetes, but I include it as an example of a diet related cause of disease.

As I was researching my condition and contemplating what I was going to have to do about It, I discovered that there was a ton of information available but that it was scattered all over the internet and in various books and magazines. I had my desktop littered with bits of information about everything and anything to do with diabetes. There was just too much to make sense of anything.

I needed to compile it into one single file that I could use as a reference. It became clear that I needed a handbook or guide book on how to reverse my diabetes. More than that I needed a user's manual on how to live a life free from diabetes. What I could and could not eat. What supplements I would need. How often I could eat and so on. That is how this book was born.

As my research progressed I came to realise what had probably caused my diabetes and what I needed to do to reverse it. It was not something that just happens apparently randomly as my first doctor had told me. There is a way out of this disease and it is not through medication.

I decided from the start that I did not want to spend the rest of my life on any medications and that would include supplements. I have since realised that in our world today supplements are a necessity and need to be included in our daily nutrition. That being said it is possible to overdose on them and most supplements work better on cyclic regimes. This is something you should consult your health advisor about.

CAUTION: DO NOT STOP TAKING YOUR MEDICATION!

I am not a doctor. Your doctor has prescribed your medications for a good reason! They control symptoms not causes. Your long term goal should be to be off medication completely but this is something you need to achieve through diet and exercise. Your doctor cannot do this for you but he can adjust your medications until you no longer need them.

Weaning yourself off medication will require regular blood testing and check-ups to monitor your requirements for the medication. As your body repairs it will no longer need medication and you run the risk of hypoglycaemia and other issues relating to overmedicating. Your doctor needs to be the person responsible for adjusting your medication. Regular appointments should include blood tests that will assist you in monitoring your progress towards better health.

My objective was to be medication free and I was willing to take risks to achieve that. I know that it is possible to do that now and I am glad that I did it. Your decisions regarding your health are your personal choices to make and I cannot make those for you.

Many people choose to stay medicated because it allows them the perceived freedom to eat a greater selection of foods. This is not a wise choice to make. Having a wider selection of poisons to choose from is not really any sort of choice at all.

Type 2 Diabetes is a lifestyle disease not a medication deficiency disease. By changing your lifestyle and quitting any bad habits you can reverse the damage that has been done and repair your body.

How long this will take will depend on how long you have had diabetes and how much damage has been done internally and how committed you are to maintaining a healthy diet and exercise program. Realistically this should be a lifetime commitment.

The simple truth is that everyone should all be eating healthier fresher foods. The lifestyles that we are leading today are the real cause of many of the illnesses that plague us. Behind the illnesses that plague us.

MY MISTAKE: I played the hero by quitting my medication and starting a new diet and fitness regime after doing only a small amount of research. I did this with only a minimum of research on diet and without consulting a dietician or healthcare professional.

The results were almost disastrous. Several factors that included the loss of a loved one, work stress and using too many supplements had me in hospital for a night with what appeared to be a heart attack! Thankfully it wasn't. My heart was fine and it was most likely just a stress reaction but it was a valuable lesson. You need to take small steps so as not to shock the body.

That being said, if your body responds really well to a new diet, then the medication could cause negative effects sooner than expected. You will need to check in regularly with your doctor to adjust your medication.

Many of the research trials done to reverse diabetes had the test subjects stop medication completely with no negative effects at all. This was done under the supervision of trained medical staff so that any changes could be noted and corrected. A Raw Vegan diet was shown to reverse diabetes in 30 days with medication being stopped within a few days of commencing the diet. Trained medical staff was constantly available to ensure that no complications happened.

Your individual case will differ from mine since I do not know how long you have had the disease or how far it has progressed. Your doctor or healthcare professional should be informed of your decision and on hand to support you if you make the commitment to stop your medication.

The healing process will take time and cannot be rushed. Your medication is there to relieve the stress on your system so that you can heal. The medication is not a cure!

The Goal is to be medication free, but the medication is an important step on the way. Taking medication when your body no longer requires it is dangerous, hence the need for regular testing and a doctor's advice on when to stop taking medication.

Consulting with your medical professional and doing regular blood tests will let you know how you are progressing and when the time is right to reduce or cease medications. Attempting to do this simply by feeling or on a whim can be disastrous.

Blood tests are a safer way to judge what is happening inside your body. They are used to track the progress of the illness so it is only fair that blood tests be used to monitor the healing process too.

Ask your doctor to arrange for blood tests that include: HbA1c, thyroid function tests, lipid Tests, liver function tests, renal function tests and a complete blood count. If you have the finances for it you might also want to have an MRI scan of your Pancreas and Liver to check their fat levels. Do this before you commence a new diet and again immediately after the diet. This should be a 25-30 day period, possibly longer if you are seriously ill.

SOME GOOD NEWS!

I am an information-junkie. I need to know stuff! I spent my childhood in libraries and in front of encyclopaedias. After I received my diagnoses, and decided to fight it, I decided to research a few cure-related news articles to keep myself motivated. The articles I found were interesting and motivational.

Professor Roy Taylor at Newcastle University conducted a study in 2011 in which 11 people, ,that all had type 2 diabetes, were put on a low calorie low carb diet for 2 months (8 weeks).[1] [2] They were limited to 600 calories per day consisting of liquid formula diet drinks and non-starchy vegetables like broccoli, cabbage and asparagus.

At the start of the study MRI scans of the patient's pancreases showed an elevated fat level of 8% where the normal level is 6%.

It is believed that excess fat in the liver and pancreas impairs the pancreas' ability to produce insulin. This fat is known as Intramyocellular Lipid. The extremely low calorie diet, with no starchy vegetables at all, prompts the body to remove fat clogging the pancreas, preventing it from making insulin.

 3 months after the study began, and the patients had returned to their normal lives, 10 of the original 11 patients were tested and 7 were still diabetes free.

MRI scans revealed that the fat levels in the pancreas had returned to normal levels and it had regained its ability to produce insulin.[3] It seems that going back to old habits undid the healing process in the other 3 patients in the study.

Below is the web address for the study with some helpful information:
http://www.ncl.ac.uk/magres/research/diabetes/reversal.htm

Professor Luke O'Neill a researcher at Trinity College and University College Dublin has discovered a protein called **Islet Amyloid Polypeptide (IAPP or Amylin)** which irritates the immune system when it occurs in the pancreas. It is believed that this may be an underlying cause for the disease.[4] IAPP is believed to have a destructive effect on cell membranes and in this way destroys the insulin producing beta cells of the pancreas.

IAPP slows down the emptying of the stomach and promotes a feeling of satiety (fullness) and thus reduces blood glucose spikes after eating a meal. IAPP is secreted with insulin from pancreatic beta cells but it appears to form deposits that destroy beta cells.

Epigallocatechin gallate (EGCG) the flavonoid found in **green tea** and **Silibinin** found in **milk thistle** have been shown to inhibit IAPP fibril formation. Tests have shown that EGCG helps to control LDL and glucose levels in the body and prevents the formation of AGEs (Advanced Glycation End products).

Milk thistle and green tea have been used for centuries in Europe and Asia to treat diabetes and kidney complaints.

Dr. Henry Daniell a molecular biologist at the University of Central Florida has genetically modified lettuce to contain the human gene code for insulin. The leaves are dried, powdered and encapsulated. When the capsules are ingested, intestinal bacteria release the insulin which stimulates an immune response and causes the body to produce its own insulin. The pancreatic beta cells started working again.

This treatment is for type 1 diabetics who cannot produce insulin but may be of use for type2 diabetics who have limited insulin production. If you are already producing insulin it may not be of any use to you especially if you are insulin resistant.

Dr. Hans Michael Dosch and **Dr Michael Salter,** researchers from The Hospital for Sick Children in Toronto, injected capsaicin into the pancreases of mice that had type 1 diabetes in an attempt to kill the animal's pain nerve cells. What happened next took them by surprise. The islet cells began producing insulin again.

The mice were no longer type 1 diabetic. It appears that malfunctioning pain nerve cells that surround the pancreas' cells prevented the islet cells from producing insulin. The nerves were not allowing enough of the neuropeptide "substance P" to be produced.

By injecting this neuropeptide into the pancreases of the mice the inflammation cleared up and the mice were no longer diabetic. The theory is that if this inflammation is treated then the pancreas can produce insulin again.

Professor Len Harrison Professor Peter Colman and Doctor Spiros Fourlanos have conducted trials proving evidence that a nasally delivered vaccine for type 1 diabetes is within reach. The researchers at Walter and Eliza Hall Institute and Royal Melbourne Hospital are working on the vaccine which is being trialled at Royal Melbourne Hospital. The trial **Intranasal Insulin Trial 11(INIT 11)** is being conducted in Australia New Zealand and Germany.[5] The vaccine works by preventing white blood cells called T cells "from attacking insulin in the pancreatic beta cells.

GLP-1 (Glucagon-like peptide-1) is a strong anti-hyperglycaemic (anti high blood sugar) hormone secreted by ileal cells in the intestine. It increases insulin secretion from the while decreasing glucagon secretion from the pancreas.

It helps to restore glucose sensitivity to pancreatic beta cells. It increases insulin sensitivity in both alpha and beta cells while also increasing the mass of pancreatic beta cells (the insulin producing cells).

It helps to promote satiety in the brain so that we do not overeat. Once in circulation it has a half-life of less than 2 minutes. In short, it tells the pancreas to make more insulin, then makes the cells more sensitive to insulin and makes us feel full after a meal so that we do not eat any more.

Melanopsin is a photoreceptive protein found in the retina which regulates circadian rhythms in mammals (i.e. the body clock). Blue light stimulates melanopsin to trigger the release of calcium which activates a gene called **NFAT** which in turn switches on other genes like **GLP-1**. It is still a very experimental theory, but it might be worth keeping an eye on.

Dr. Gabriel Cousens founder of The Tree of life Oasis in Arizona took six volunteers and put them on a raw vegan organic diet for thirty days. They were asked to stop taking their medication for the duration of the thirty days. The results were all the same. No More Medication Required! The full story is available as a documentary called ***"Simply Raw: Reversing Diabetes in 30 Days"*** which chronicles their cure.

You can watch a promo video on YouTube by searching for ***"Simply Raw: Reversing Diabetes in 30 Days"*** **www.gabrielcousens.com.**

Patrick Holford has had success in reversing diabetes in patients by using a low GI / GL diet with supplements and exercise.   **www.patrickholford.com**

Dr. Fedon Lindberg a Norwegian endocrinologist practising from both Norway and Greece has had success in reversing diabetes. He prescribes a Low Glycaemic Index (GI) and Low Glycaemic load (GL) Mediterranean style diet. Unprocessed fruits, vegetables, pulses, grains and extra virgin olive oil are staples of the diet. **www.drlindberg.com**

Dr. Neal Barnard has reversed diabetes in patients by putting them on a vegan diet that includes starchy carbs, exercise and supplements. He advocates a low fat vegetarian diet that contains little to no vegetable oils and absolutely no animal products at all. It is essentially a plant based diet and there are no restrictions on how much you can eat. **www.nealbarnard.org**

DeWayne McCulley has cured himself of diabetes and written a book detailing everything necessary for you to do

the same. He survived a diabetes related coma and came back fighting and determined to be cured. It is an incredibly detailed and in-depth book with solid scientific information to back up the recommendations.
www.deathtodiabetes.com

Dr. Joel Fuhrman has had success in reversing diabetes with his dietary approach to health. He is a medical doctor who has taken a dietary approach to curing patients rather than drug therapy approach. He is also seen in the documentary film: **"Fat, Sick and Nearly Dead"** which chronicles the journey of Joe Cross from fat and unhealthy to healthy by doing a juice fast.
www.drfuhrman.com

http://www.rebootwithjoe.com/about/fat-sick-and-nearly-dead/

Dr. Stefan Ripich and Jim Healthy Dr. Stefan Ripich is a naturopathic physician who has had success in reversing patients' diabetes with a diet that has an emphasis on raw foods. He has teamed up with Jim Healthy to create a dietary program to reverse diabetes.
www.30daydiabetescure.com

Gastric bypass, lap-band surgery, Stomach Stapling all known as **Bariatric Surgery** have been shown to reverse the symptoms of type 2 diabetes.

These are just a small handful of the articles and people I discovered during my research there are many more.

There are many other doctors and other medical professionals who have taken the position that diabetes is reversible rather than just treatable.

Not all doctors are on board with this opinion, however, so choose your doctor for his positive attitude rather than his skills as a drug pusher. Doctors are also businessmen after all and we cannot blame them for wanting to earn a living.

There is a growing population of ex-diabetics out there. These are people who have had diabetes and are now free of diabetes. There are more than a few documented cases of people who have reversed their diabetes by following strict diets without the need for any medication. Diet is the single most important factor in achieving a reversal of this disease. Halle Berry and Drew Carey are 2 of the more famous diabetic cases that have reversed their symptoms.

A diet that is low in fat low in GI / GL and focusses on vegetables is a recurring theme in all the success stories. There are also a few key supplements that diabetics are prone to being deficient in. Supplementing with these will assist in the reversal of the disease.

Many people choose not to change their diet and rely on the medication to keep them going. The problem with this attitude is that it only masks the damage. The damage is still there. Underneath it is starting to decay but it is invisible until it's too late. It is like painting over rust. Medication slows down the decay but it does not stop it or reverse it and as time progresses you will need more medication.

The body is designed to be self-healing but if we do not feed it with the necessary nutrients to do this then we cannot expect it to heal. I have changed what I eat. I have changed how I eat. I have stopped taking any medication at all. I have medical tests that prove I no longer have type 2 diabetes the very same tests that were used to diagnose me as a type 2 diabetic. I know this is possible because I have done it and now I have proof and continue to get tested to add to my proof.

Changing your diet will have a profoundly positive effect on your health and state of mind. This may sound easy but it is the most difficult change you will ever make in your life. It is for this reason so many people choose to rely on medication rather than change a lifetimes' worth of bad habits. It is a decision that will affect you at least 3 times a day, every day. It will affect you every time you go out socially.

My first doctor told me that the disease would get progressively worse that there was no cure or reversal and that I had to take all those pills and make a few changes to my diet.

He told me that it would get worse over time and gave me a few of the diabetic issues to look forward to like amputation and blindness. You may have heard this already from your doctor.

I felt as though I was being sent off to die and that pissed me off!

 I refuse to accept not having a choice!

There are always choices we are just not always aware of them. I have made myself aware of these choices.

The fact that you are holding this book and reading this paragraph means that you too are now aware that you have choices. The next step is to make a choice.

JONATHAN PRINS

Auckland New Zealand, May 2012

Follow us on:

Website: **www.krazykea.com**

BlogSpot: **www.krazykeapublishing.blogspot.com**

Facebook: **Cure diabetes naturally**

 Youtube:
http://www.youtube.com/user/krazykeapublishing

Twitter: **Krazy_kea**

DIABETES:
THE BASICS

A BRIEF HISTORY OF DIABETES

The earliest report of diabetes was in 1550BC in an Egyptian papyrus. It spoke of rapid weight loss and frequent urination in patients and is believed to be the first written reference to diabetes. It is not known whether this was type 1 or type 2 diabetes.

During the middle ages the Arabian physician Avicenna detailed the progress and complications of the disease.

By the early 19th Century chemical test were devised to detect high sugar content in urine. During this time the French physician Bouchardat discovered that a calorie restricted diet was beneficial to his diabetic patients.

More recently researchers have discovered that insulin was produced by both the pancreas *and* the brain. They determined that a drop in brain produced insulin contributes to a degeneration of brain cells which is an early symptom of Alzheimer's.

Alzheimer's patients have impaired insulin production in their brains. They discovered that insulin and IGF 1(insulin-like growth factor) were significantly reduced in the frontal cortex, hippocampus and hypothalamus. These are all areas of the brain affected by the progression of Alzheimer's.

The theory is that Alzheimer's disease could be seen to be type of diabetes. It has even been called type 3 diabetes, although this name has not stuck. Insulin resistance prevents brain cells from using glucose as the primary fuel resulting in the death of brain cells.

Ketones appear to be an acceptable alternative fuel source for the brain cells and have shown to slow the progression of Alzheimer's and even reverse some of the symptoms. Ketones are metabolised in the liver after the consumption of **medium chain triglycerides (MCT's)** like those found in coconut oil.

INSULIN

Much has been said about the dangers of high blood glucose levels but no-one mentions the dangers of high insulin levels. While insulin is vitally important there is a danger in having high insulin levels particularly in the case of insulin resistance.

When your cells are insulin resistant your body produces more insulin to force the glucose into the cells. This results in high blood levels of insulin. Insulin is also a storage hormone that encourages the storage of fats.

High insulin levels will take up to 25% of all ingested calories and turn them into fat regardless of how much or how little you eat. This convinces your body into thinking that you are starving which means that you feel hungry, regardless of how much you eat, and that you feel tired and lethargic all the time. To the outside world you simply appear lazy and gluttonous.

Fructose is the leading cause behind this. It is processed by the liver but does not need insulin to regulate it. It does however cause insulin resistance in the liver and also raises total body insulin levels and 30% of all fructose ingested will be stored as fat.

Avoiding sugar, fructose, high fructose corn syrup (HFCS), honey, agave syrup, maple syrup, fruit juice and any of the other "safe" or "natural" sugars is the only way to reset the insulin balance since they all contain fructose.

Whole fruit is the only sweet treat acceptable since the fibre content slows down the rate at which fructose is metabolised.

Whole fruit is also not a concentrated source of fructose like fruit juice would be (1 glass of apple juice is worth about 10-12 apples without the benefit of fibre).

WHAT IS TYPE 2 DIABETES?

Diabetes is a chronic disorder of the protein, fat and carbohydrate metabolism. It is characterized by high fasting levels of blood glucose. High blood glucose levels are also responsible for frequent urination (polyuria) and increased thirst (polydipsia), chronic inflammation and blurred vision. What you eat, physical stress and psychological stress all have the ability to raise blood sugar levels.

When you eat food your body turns that food into glucose. The trillions of cells in your body all use glucose as their fuel. The glucose is absorbed through the small intestine into the capillaries and into the bloodstream. Some of the glucose is stored in the liver to be used as a backup supply such as between meals or during sleeping or fasting.

As the blood glucose levels rise after a meal, the pancreas senses the glucose and releases the hormone insulin. Insulin "unlocks" the cells so that glucose can enter them and be used as fuel. Unfortunately for some of us our cells become immune to insulin and the pancreas releases more insulin to try to "force" the glucose into the cells.

Small amounts of fat, called Lipid Droplets or Intramyocellular Lipids clog up the cell wall preventing the insulin from opening the cell membrane to allow the glucose in. This Intramyocellular fat is one of the contributors of insulin resistance.

As the insulin resistance gets worse the pancreas has to pump out enormous amounts of insulin to get the same amount of glucose into the cells. If the condition remains untreated the insulin-producing beta cells in the pancreas burn out and stop working and you are forced to give yourself daily insulin injections to stay alive.

WHAT CAUSES TYPE 2 DIABETES?

In 2007 researchers at The University of California San Diego (UCSD) School of Medicine discovered that inflammation provoked by immune cells called macrophages contributes to insulin resistance and Type 2 Diabetes.[6]

MACROPHAGES: are found in white blood cells and bone marrow and play a very important part in the immune response. They function as both specific and non-specific defence mechanisms. They are phagocytes (cell-devouring) cells that attack foreign substances, infectious microbes and cancer cells. Macrophages accumulate in people with type 2 diabetes and cause diabetic complications such as neuropathy, nephropathy, retinopathy and atherosclerosis. When macrophages get into tissue such as adipose (fat) or liver tissue they release cytokines.

CYTOKINES: are cell-signalling proteins (chemical messenger molecules), secreted by the glial cells of the immune system and nervous system for intercellular communication. They help regulate the body's response to disease and infection. They target and bind with immune cells and this triggers a specific response from the immune cells.

Overproduction of cytokines however can actually cause disease. Cytokines cause the liver muscle or fat cells to become insulin resistant or diabetic. Cytokines secreted by adipose (fat) tissue directly affects insulin secretion.

ADIPONECTINS: are cytokines that are inversely related to body fat, i.e. thin people will have high levels of adiponectins and obese people will have low levels of adiponectins. It is believed that low levels of adiponectins may cause hyperinsulinemia (high insulin levels).

There are theories about toxins like **alloxan** (a by-product of the bleaching process in white flour production) and **bisphenol-A** (a constituent in some plastics) as being the cause of diabetes. There may be some truth in these allegations since alloxan is used to artificially induce diabetes (called alloxan diabetes) in lab animals.

The common factors in diabetes, however, remain the same: obesity, sedentary lifestyles and poor diet seem to be the cornerstones for building a life plagued by diabetes. Consuming too much processed food will stimulate an inflammatory response from the immune system.

In 1993 scientists discovered a gene they called **FABP2**.They were studying the Pima Indians who have the highest prevalence of type 2 diabetes in any ethnic group in the world. There had not been any instances of diabetes amongst this particular ethnic group before. It is believed that the sudden change from traditional agricultural foods to modern processed foods is what contributed to the high prevalence of diabetes amongst the Pima Indians.

It seems that the gene FABP2 is responsible for making threonine an amino acid which creates an intestinal fatty acid binding protein. When the gene makes the protein the body absorbs more fatty acids from fat in food. This leads to a higher level of fat and fatty acids in the blood which contributes towards insulin resistance.

THE STORY OF THE PIMA INDIANS

In the 1870's the U.S. government diverted the river that was the Pima's primary source of water for crops and fishing which led to a forty year drought. When the U.S Federal government finally stepped in to assist the Pima it was only to supply them with canned and processed foods.

They were supplied with food that would last a while without spoiling since their original means of gathering food had been taken away.
Changing their diets from traditional grains, fish, game and vegetables to western processed foods removing the need to do any traditional work activities combined with a gene code whose purpose was to extract more fatty acids from food (a survival gene called FABP2) has not been a good transition for this ethnic group.

Their new diet was mostly canned, processed foods, sugar and flour. A diet high in starchy carbohydrates and saturated fats combined with a gene code that extracts more fatty acids from food particularly when those fatty acids are the unhealthy ones proved fatally dangerous for this ethnic population.

They were much less physically active since their primary activities of hunting and farming were now replaced by opening a can of corned beef. Their diet was now high fat, low fibre and high carbohydrate.

INTRAMYOCELLULAR LIPIDS: are microscopic fat droplets that clog up the inside of cells. They make cells inflexible and impermeable. They prevent insulin from opening up the cells to allow glucose in. A diet high in fat, particularly animal fat, is the leading cause of this.

If you were to check the WHO statistics for which countries top the list for diabetes you would notice an alarming trend amongst them. They all have starchy, processed white carbohydrates as staples in their diet! These countries have also had significant changes occur in their food sources.

There are now more animal fats, vegetable oils and sugars than there were traditionally and also more processed foods and drinks. The countries topping the diabetes list are India, China, America, Russia, Indonesia, Japan and Pakistan.

These countries have had their traditional diets changed to adapt to a modern world and not necessarily a western one. Their diets now contain processed foods with high levels of sucrose and fructose, which were not available decades ago.

Traditional grains have been processed and stripped of all fibre and nutrition, leaving only starch behind. The way these foods are processed, has also changed, to suit modern production and preservation standards.

As ethnic cultures have modernised, they have lost some of their traditional way of doing things in favour of technology and commerce. Traditional fats have been replaced by "heart friendly" fats. Wholegrain flour has been replaced by refined and bleached flour. Fruit juices are now easily available where they were not before as with candies and confectionary.

A lot has been said about the "western" diet being the culprit behind many diseases, but clearly this is not the case in diabetes. It seems to be a "modern" lifestyle that is affecting us all. Our lives may be busier than ever but our activity levels are lower. Our diets now contain more saturated animal fats than ever before. Refrigeration, transportation and preservation methods have made available to us, on a daily basis, food items that were only consumed occasionally or at special events. The nutritional quality of our food is now of less importance than its shelf-life and its profit margin.
At some point, something had to happen and I believe that type 2 diabetes is that something.

It is not how much we eat but what we eat! (This is not permission to go for gold at the buffet table, however, since overeating leads to weight gain and increases the risk of developing diabetes).

The consumption of fatty foods with starchy, high carbohydrate foods, sugar, fructose, large amounts of animal protein and a sedentary lifestyle all contribute towards getting diabetes and there is no cultural or time barrier on that!

Consuming foods with a high glycemic value and taking in too much sugar are the underlying causes for diabetes. Excess calories stored as fat, paired with continuously high

blood glucose levels, causes the various metabolic processes that lead to the condition called type 2 diabetes mellitus.

HOW DO YOU GET TYPE 2 DIABETES?

Diabetes is a "lifestyle disease" and several lifestyle factors
are involved in developing diabetes. It is NOT genetic.
You get it by following the examples set by your parents or
role models. These are lifestyle choices not genetic codes.

Diabetes was once called a disease of affluence meaning
that only wealthy people once got it. These were people
who could eat lavish, fatty, sweet meals and did not do
physical labour and had access to foods that were refined
and expensive.

This is no longer the case. We all have access to refined
foods and various other processed foods today and who
needs exercise when you have television!

Refined, processed foods, animal proteins and fats and refined carbohydrates like sugar and fructose are in everything we see on supermarket shelves.

Here are a few of the basics in the recipe to developing diabetes:

1. **Exercising** too little if ever at all. A sedentary lifestyle will slow down your metabolism and lead to weight gain. Energy is stored rather than used.
2. **Excessive** intake of saturated animal fats like those found in beef and lamb and dairy products like milk, butter and cheese. This leads to weight gain when too many carbohydrates are consumed as well.
3. **Stress:** raises your adrenal hormones like epinephrine (adrenaline) and cortisol which raises blood glucose levels and makes you insulin resistant. It also causes poor sleep patterns cravings for "junk" foods and the potential for stimulant abuse. It also wears out the organs responsible for making these hormones.
4. **Stimulants:** abuse of stimulants such as caffeine, nicotine and alcohol which raise blood pressure and blood glucose levels and damages arteries.
5. **Insufficient** intake of omega-3 oils for cell repair and good brain functioning along with omega-6 fatty acids.
6. **Insufficient** intake of vegetables, particularly leafy greens, which contain phytonutrients and anti-oxidants needed for repair and detoxing.
7. **Fructose and Sucrose** this is by far the biggest cause of type 2 diabetes. By drinking too many sodas and fruit juices, eating too many sweet treats and many other foods that have "hidden" sugar in them, like ice

lollies, bottled sauces, syrups and jams, all of which stimulate fatty deposits in the liver and pancreas and cause insulin resistance.

Sugar has also been proven to be as addictive as some opioid drugs, affecting the same areas of the brain as these opioid drugs. If you find it hard to give up sugar it is most likely because you are addicted to it.

8. **Excessive intake of Carbohydrate:** dietary "staples" like white rice, white flour, bread, pasta, breakfast cereals and anything made from these, in fact, stay away from any white foods, including vegetables like potato and parsnip. Starchy carbohydrates raise blood glucose and blood insulin levels very quickly. This promotes fat storage if the calories are not burned up during exercise, not to mention the other negative side effects of high levels of glucose and insulin such as inflammation.

By the time you are diagnosed as type 2 diabetic, the damage is already done; the question is only how much damage has been done. In some cases, people have been diabetic for years before being diagnosed. If you are diagnosed as pre-diabetic, it means that you are on the road to doing damage but can still change direction before it is too late.

Most people have already gone past pre-diabetes without even knowing about it, since diabetes does not cause any pain or discomfort at the start. Reversal of the damage is difficult. It will require willpower and commitment, but it can be done!

There is an abundance of scientific proof for this. You just need resolve and commitment.

MY STORY

My wife and I immigrated to another country. We sold the house packed up our belongings, shipped the dog over, said goodbye to our friends and family and off we went. A requirement of the Immigration process is a full medical check-up. I had blood tests, urine tests, x-rays and then some. I had them done twice, with a six month break between each set of tests. I was pronounced healthy i.e. **not diabetic!**

All of this took place in the middle of the global economic recession and work was not easy to come by. I took a job at the local butchers shop, as I had recently done training in butchery, to add to my chef skills. The entire process was all a little stressful but nothing too hard to handle, so where did it all go wrong?

Here's what happened:

I found myself working for a businessman who was incompetent. I worked for someone who married into a wealthy family that bought him a business that he had no ability to run.

His position as a manager had been purchased through nepotism and not earned through skill or ability. He was very frustrating to work for. His ego was behind many poor decisions both moral and financial.

For four years, I found myself working 10-16 hours a day, sometimes longer, in a poorly managed work environment. There was no leadership, no organisation and no accountability, whatsoever. The work environment was unorganised, unprofessional and often unethical.

Having worked and trained in both butchery and as a chef, I found myself being told to do things I knew to be wrong but was unable to correct. I soon learned not to argue with someone who always knew better than anyone else but it was frustrating and demotivating.

My choices were to either do things that I knew to be wrong or risk getting fired. These were tough choices for an immigrant to make during a recession, when unfamiliar with a different culture. I made the wrong choice and stayed on.

I allowed myself to be exposed to stress every day for four years, thinking I was handling it, certain that I was coping with it. At some point I began to experience frequent eye twitches and headaches and would become irritable and easily angered. I did not think much of these symptoms at the time, considering them to be minor stress related issues and supplemented with vitamin B complex, which I had heard, was good for that. But things were happening internally slowly and without any noticeable pain or discomfort.

I thought I could ignore the warnings, but I was wrong. I was beginning to get stressed and like most people, I was not aware that I was becoming stressed.

I soon lost the motivation to do any physical activity because I was too physically and mentally exhausted at the end of the day to even think, let alone exercise. I had very minimal control over my personal time because there was absolutely no organisation in my work schedule. This meant that I was unable to plan ahead for anything in my life outside of work because I had no set schedule. Knock-off time was whenever the boss decided.

10-16 hour long work days meant that I was not getting enough sleep either. I was fatigued, tired and lethargic all the time. I was urinating frequently too, but put this down to the caffeine in the numerous energy drinks I was consuming.

Since my wife and I both worked, there was nobody at home to prepare nutritious meals. We found ourselves eating take-out more often than not. Take-out was cheap and tasted good and you don't have to do dishes when you are done eating at 9:30pm and are too tired to even stand upright. Lunches were sandwiches, meat pies, greasy take-outs or more meat again, since I worked in butchery.

Sweet treats, pastries and candy bars were also regular additions to meals as comfort foods that made me feel better (I was addicted to sugar without knowing it). I would occasionally eat fruit with my lunch and somehow concluded that this made me "healthy". I would also replace diet soda and energy drinks with fruit juice, drinking up to a litre a day, since I hated the taste of water, thinking the juice was healthy. I was wrong. This was a near fatal mistake; I did not know what the consequence of regular fructose consumption was.

Having been a chef before, you would think I knew better but yet somehow none of this registered as dangerous. I did not yet physically feel ill, so I did not think anything was wrong. Stress hormones affect the food choices we make. I know this now.

Working in a butchery meant access to lots of meat. I was eating a lot of red meat (steak is tasty and cooks quickly) and processed meats. I convinced myself that the iron and protein in red meat was good for me. As long as I didn't eat the fat, I would not have cholesterol issues, choosing to forget that red meat has fat in the muscle and that **all** animal protein has cholesterol. Again I was wrong. The unhealthier I became, the dumber I became and the better I got at justifying my poor choices.

I had never liked the taste of water and would drink diet soda, sports electrolytes and fruit juice to stay hydrated. I told myself that they were made with water and that was good enough. I chose to ignore the fact that I was placing my liver and kidneys under immense pressure, by forcing them to process all that garbage! These beverages have sugars, salts, chemicals and food acids in them that completely upset the PH of the body. The fructose was going straight to my liver, to be turned into fat by the truckload.

As my diet grew progressively worse, I started to feel more lethargic, run down and exhausted. Thank god there were cheap, sugar-laden, caffeine spiked energy drinks to keep me going! Caffeine, sugar and refined carbohydrates were my fuel.

Four years into the job, I found myself sitting in a doctor's office, shell-shocked, feeling like I'd just been punched in the face, with my wife in tears beside me. I had just been diagnosed with type 2 diabetes!

I felt like I had been hit by a freight train. Diabetes was something other people got not me. I was too young for this. Diabetes is hereditary isn't it? I have no family history of this disease! How does this happen?

My doctor at the time told me it just happens and that it was irreversible and that it would get progressively worse. Don't worry about it, we have pills for you. You may have heard similar words.

I had told the manager I would be a few minutes late that morning, as I had a doctor's appointment and when I got to work that morning, looking like I'd seen a ghost, the manager smiling and gleefully clapping his hands together, asked if I had cancer and if I was going to die. This event actually happened; I do not include it for dramatic effect. Maybe he meant it as a joke, maybe not.

Either way, it was a pivotal moment for me. For the second time that morning, I felt like I had been face-punched. It was turning out to be my worst day ever. I took it personally and decided that this was going to be a battle I would fight.

I could now visualise an opponent for whom I did not have to show any mercy. Diabetes had become a personal matter and I would cure myself of it or die trying! If diabetes was going to kill me anyway then I had nothing to lose and everything to gain by trying.

Visualization is a powerful psychological tool. Mind controls matter and if we can control our minds we can control our bodies. Visualising your opponent losing is an important psychological aspect of any battle. See yourself destroying this disease in whatever way suits you personally, so long as you see yourself winning

It's not a Brussels sprout; it's a hand grenade in the war against diabetes!

Now I cannot blame an incompetent manager for the garbage that I put into my body, nor can I blame him for my decision not to exercise. Those were my choices and I have to live with the consequences of them. I blame no-one but myself. So why am I whining?

Answer: I have learned that the people around me can have a dramatic impact on my peace of mind and consequently my health. We often find ourselves in situations that stress us. Other people will have an impact on our time and our state of mind if we allow them to.

These situations need to be resolved. Apply enough pressure and you can crack a diamond. We sometimes have people in our lives that are either actively or passively detrimental to us physically and/or psychologically.

Our bodies are not immune to this. We find ways to relieve the pressure and too often this means food. We overeat, emotional eat and reward ourselves with food. In small doses, spaced far apart, this may not cause any problems but when done on a daily basis, this leads to disease.

Psychologically and physiologically, we crave foods that are harmful to us in the long term. It's a stress response that makes us crave foods that will be stored for energy in the face of impending danger. Stress hormones cause us to crave these types of foods. Sugar affects the reward centre of the brain so we eat sweet things and get a "happy" high from it. If you keep treating yourself to sweet things when you feel stressed it is only a matter of time before something goes wrong.

Sugar has been shown to affect opioid receptors in the brain. This implies that sugar has addictive properties just like heroin or morphine. You are addicted to sugar without knowing it!

Dopamine stimulates the reward centre of the brain. This is where drug addicts get their high from. Sugar affects these dopamine receptors in the same way that it does for people on hard drugs. Eventually tolerance will build up and you will need more sugar to get the same high. This is addiction. Sugar is addictive and unlike hard drugs, you can get it at the grocery store!

Your happiness and your health are inextricably linked. I thought I was able to withstand the stress of dealing with an incompetent, egotistical, dishonest "leader" but I was wrong. I was unhappy and soon became unwell by making the wrong choice/s.

Eating was my crutch and putting garbage into my system was my reward for having to endure my daily dose of stress. I spent more time relaxing and being sedentary and justified this by telling myself that I deserved to relax. Big surprise I got diabetes!

These were my coping mechanisms. Others may find themselves turning to alcohol or substance abuse. The ways in which we abuse ourselves are as numerous as we are. Become aware of what you are doing to yourself.

Stress is a killer. It comes disguised innocuously as events or people we know, like an incompetent egotistical boss in my case. You may have different types of stressors in your life or you may have none at all.

The people and situations in your life need to be examined and evaluated to find out which of them are leading you to make the wrong choices. There is a proven connection between poor eating habits and depression and disease. The difficulty lies in being aware of what is happening.

For some it might not be a person or event but apathy or a lack of direction or even boredom. It took me 4 years to wake up and understand what was going wrong.

In our lives we are going to encounter people or situations that raise our blood pressure. It is natural and unavoidable. In small doses it is even healthy. Prolonged exposure to stress however causes changes in our physical and psychological makeup. In a later chapter I will discuss what stress does to the body and techniques on how to relieve it.

Type 2 diabetes is a physical bodily reaction to a change in our psychology and diet. If we can change our psychology then we can change our physiology. Our diet is another matter.

There are several theories that suggest a connection between disease and agriculture. As we have discovered how to make our food more readily available, concentrated and processed, we have also become subjected to new diseases.

ECONOMIC FACTORS OF DIABETES

Stress is not the only cause for disease. Poverty is another strong reason. Ever noticed how the foods that are bad for you are cheap and the foods that are good for you are expensive. Is it any wonder then why so many people are ill when a large part of their daily nutrition comes from junk food? Fast food chains have cheap tasty meal deals that are hard to ignore when you don't have much money.

Processed foods are generally cheaper than wholefoods. They have extended shelf lives and are cheap, tasty and easy to prepare, if any preparation at all is required. The trouble with processed foods is that they are loaded with sugars, salts, fats and chemicals designed to increase shelf-life and palatability.

There is not much consideration for health and nutrition even when such claims are made. Something might be low in fat but high in fructose. Added vitamins and minerals are used as selling points to mask the fact that all the original nutrients were stripped away during processing.

Processed food manufacturers compete with each other for customers and the result is foods that are cheaper and tastier but unhealthier. It is a battle of company profits vs. consumer health.Eating healthy is going to cost you a little more, but you can either spend the money on healthy food or you can spend it on medical bills. One way or another, the money will get spent, you get to choose how. What is the price tag on your health?

A WESTERN DISEASE

The WHO statistics for countries with a growing diabetes rate shows an alarming trend common to them all. They all have starchy, processed white carbohydrates as staples in their diet! These countries have also had significant changes occur in their food sources over the past several decades.

There are now more saturated animal fats and refined carbohydrates, processed foods, and fructose laden soft drinks available. India, China, America, Russia, Indonesia, Japan and Pakistan have all succumbed to this "western" disease.

As these countries have adapted to modern food production methods, their diets have changed accordingly. There is more sucrose and fructose, trans-fats and saturated fats available from many sources. Traditional grains have been processed and stripped of all fibre and nutrition leaving only starch behind, in other words, a high glycaemic and high fat diet.

As ethnic cultures have modernised they have lost some of their traditional way of doing things in favour of technology and commerce. There is less physical activity to burn off stored energy.

Traditional fats have been replaced by "heart friendly" fats which have upset the omega-3 / omega-6 fatty acid balance. The belief that "It's healthy so you can eat more" has created an imbalance in our diets.

Wholegrain flour has been replaced by refined and bleached flour. Fruit juices are now available where they were not before and the same with candies and confectionary. Packaged processed foods are easily available and convenient. We are losing our health for the sake of convenience.

A lot has been said about the "western" diet being the culprit to many diseases but clearly this is not the case in diabetes. It seems to be a "modern" lifestyle that is affecting us all. The terms "western" and "modern" are not the same. Our lives may be busier than ever but our activity levels are less than ever before.

Our diets have more saturated animal fats than ever before. Refrigeration transportation and preservation methods have made available to us on daily basis foods that were only consumed occasionally or at special events. The nutritional quality of our food is now of less importance than its shelf-life and its profit margin.

We have access to foods now in quantities unheard of before. Our foods are available all year round; there is no real seasonal aspect to our foods anymore.

Almost every industrialised culture on this planet is now consuming foods to excess. We have choices about what to eat and we only choose what we like. These choices are not always the best for us.

At some point something had to happen and I believe that type 2 diabetes is that something. The problem is just as much what we eat as it is how much we eat.

The consumption of fatty foods with starchy high carbohydrate foods, sugar, fructose, large amounts of animal protein and a sedentary lifestyle all contribute towards getting diabetes and there is no cultural or time barrier on that!

This is not a "western" disease, it is a "modern" disease that is caused by modern food production techniques and the overabundance of fructose and Trans saturated fats in our processed foods along with much more sedentary lifestyles.

CHROMIUM

This essential mineral is partly responsible for the metabolism of proteins, fats and carbohydrates. Unfortunately, it is stripped from grains and other foods when being refined into the "food" that sits on supermarket shelves. Many nutrients are stripped from our foods during processing and that is why so many packaging containers have the words "fortified with added vitamins and minerals" printed on them.

Insulin requires a receptor to work properly. Chromium increases the number of receptors and helps insulin bind stronger to those receptors. It enhances the effect of insulin. Most of us are deficient in chromium and are not aware of it, diabetics in particular. Chromium also helps to relieve depression, lower cholesterol and blood lipids, to decrease body fat and increase lean body mass.

There are 2 supplements available: chromium picolinate and chromium polynicotinate.

Chromium polynicotinate is chelated with niacin (vitamin B3)

Nicotinic acid, vitamin PP and picolinate are bound to tryptophan to create **chromium picolinate**.

There are reports that picolinate causes chromosomal damage in large doses, whereas polynicotinate appears to be safe in similar doses.

DIABETES: CONSEQUENCES

"The superior doctor prevents sickness; the mediocre doctor attends to impending sickness; the inferior doctor treats actual sickness;"

- Chinese proverb

In 2011, the World health organization (WHO) reported that there were 346 million known cases of diabetes in the world. This figure is only an estimate, as it does not include those who have not yet been tested, whether living in first or third world countries. More cases are added daily.

It has also been suggested that up to 25% of the world population, has some degree of insulin resistance or a type of metabolic issue. With a world population of 7 billion in 2012 that would mean that 1in every 4 people either has or may soon have type 2 diabetes or some form of metabolic syndrome.

Left unchecked, diabetes can damage the heart, blood vessels, eyes, kidneys, pancreas and nerves over time. It increases the risk of heart disease and stroke. Up to 50% of people with diabetes die of cardiovascular disease or stroke. They suffer from many diabetes related issues before this happens.

The big question is: How did Type 2 Diabetes become such a plague, almost overnight?

I believe that our bodies are unable to process the concentrated and refined "foods" that we are eating. These foods exist in abundance today, where they were less plentiful decades ago.

Diabetes is more than just "a little sugar problem". There are a number of serious conditions waiting for you if you leave it untreated or unmanaged.

DIABETIC CARDIOMYOPATHY (HEART DISEASE)

Coronary Heart Disease (CHD), heart failure and diabetic cardiomyopathy are potential diseases awaiting diabetics.

CHD occurs when plaque builds up in the arteries reducing blood flow. This causes pain (angina), irregular heartbeats (arrhythmias), heart attacks and death. Heart failure occurs when the heart cannot pump enough blood to meet the body's needs.

Diabetic cardiomyopathy is diagnosed when there is damage to the structure and function of the heart. The heart is unable to properly circulate blood throughout the body and there is a fluid build-up in the lungs and or legs. Heart failure is the end result of untreated cardiomyopathy. It is diagnosed when there are no signs of coronary artery disease as the two diseases are very different.

In cardiomyopathy the heart muscle changes under the influence of stress hormones or untreated continuous high blood sugar levels. The heart muscle thickens or forms scar tissue and is less able to do its job properly.

Exercise, diet, reducing stress, managing blood glucose and blood cholesterol will all help prevent this heart disease, but there are very few treatments for it. Stem cell therapy or the fitting of a pacemaker are the most common solutions.

High blood levels of **homocysteine** and **C-reactive protein** are all markers for heart disease, so ask your doctor to do regular blood tests for these. These are made worse in the presence of high blood pressure so try to keep your blood pressure under control too.

Diabetic cardiomyopathy is an intricate and complicated disease with some differences to "conventional" heart disease but the causes and treatments are similar with the focus on lowering blood glucose levels. Diet and aerobic exercise are the best solution to maintain a healthy heart.

Heart disease is believed to be related to insulin resistance. High levels of insulin will distort the balance of "good" HDL vs. "bad" LDL cholesterol in the blood. High blood glucose levels allow for Glycation reactions to occur. Glycation occurs when a protein or fat joins with a sugar.

When LDL cholesterol joins with blood glucose it forms *Glycated LDL* which is easily oxidized and damages **endothelial nitric oxide synthase** an enzyme needed to maintain proper vasodilation and blood flow. *Glycated LDL* is not recognised by LDL receptors on cell surfaces and remains in circulation contributing towards atherosclerosis.

DIABETIC NEUROPATHY

Neuropathy is damage caused to the small blood vessels that supply nerves as a result of diabetes and affects up to 50% of people with diabetes. Although many different problems can occur as a result of diabetic neuropathy common symptoms are tingling, pain, numbness or weakness in the feet and hands, facial drooping, erectile dysfunction, incontinence, involuntary muscle contraction, dizziness and burning or pain sensations, combined with reduced blood flow, neuropathy in the feet increases the chance of foot ulcers and wounds leading to serious infections and eventual limb amputation.

ALA (alpha-lipoic acid) in doses of 600mg-1800mg per day and B12 (Methylcobalimin) have proven very effective in treating neuropathy. Make certain that you do not confuse alpha-linolenic acid (an omega-3 fatty acid) with alpha-lipoic acid (an antioxidant) as the two are both often abbreviated as ALA.

Nicotine is a vasoconstrictor (shrinks blood vessels) and should be avoided at all costs in all delivery formats including patches and electronic cigarettes. Quit now!

DIABETIC RETINOPATHY

Retinopathy is a leading cause of blindness and occurs as a result of long-term accumulated damage to the small blood vessels in the retina. After 15 years of diabetes approximately 2% of people become blind and about 10% develop severe visual impairment.

Poorly controlled blood glucose, high blood pressure and cholesterol along with smoking are all risk factors for developing retinopathy. There are treatments to prevent vision loss but once damage has occurred it is not reversible.

Manage your blood glucose levels, blood pressure levels and blood cholesterol now to avoid losing your sight in the future. And again quit, smoking now!

DIABETIC NEPHROPATHY (KIDNEY DISEASE)

Diabetes related nephropathy is one of the leading causes of kidney failure with 10-20% of diabetics dying of kidney failure. Each kidney is made up of hundreds of thousands of tiny structures called nephrons. These nephrons filter the blood and remove waste from the body. Poor blood glucose control and high blood pressure cause damage to the kidneys. The nephrons thicken and form scar tissue. The kidneys begin to leak and albumin (protein) passes into the urine. Because the kidneys are no longer working correctly there now toxins in the blood and dialysis may be needed to remove them.

Have your urine checked for high levels of protein as this is an indicator of kidney damage. Smoking raises the risk for kidney damage. Blood glucose control, blood pressure control, diet and regular exercise all help prevent kidney damage.

URIC ACID

High levels of uric acid in the blood are often associated with diabetes. This can lead to gout and kidney stones if left unchecked and may also cause kidney disease in not treated. It may in fact be a symptom of the kidneys not working properly or it may be diet related.

Uric acid is a by-product of the breakdown of compounds called purines that are present in some food sources.

Brewer's yeast, baker's yeast, herring, mackerel, tuna, salmon, scallops, anchovies, sardines, sweetbreads, liver beef kidneys, brains and most organ meats, meat extracts like Oxo and Bovril, game meats and gravy are all foods that are high in purines.

Dried peas, lentils, beans, oatmeal, wheat bran and wheat germ are vegetable sources that also contain moderate amounts of purines. Diets that are connected to gout have been shown to be similar to those of people with cardio-vascular disease. Animal research has shown that rats fed a diet with a 10% uric acid content will develop diabetes.

MY MISTAKE: I decided to use pea derived vegetable protein in my breakfast smoothies rather than whey or soy protein. Only after getting a blood test result with a high uric acid level did I discover that peas have a high purine content which is greatly increased when used as a protein isolate supplement. I stopped using it and everything re-turned to normal.

The body uses potassium, sodium, magnesium, calcium and zinc to neutralize high uric acid levels in the system which means a greater potential for deficiencies in these minerals if you have high uric acid levels. Make sure that you are taking a good quality multivitamin supplement containing these minerals. Drinking decaffeinated coffee has been shown to cause a modest decrease in uric acid levels in the blood.

Colourful vegetables and vegetable juices are low in purines. Try adding things like cucumber, celery, beetroot radish, carrots, leafy greens, capsicum, red cabbage and tomatoes to your diet and drink plenty of filtered water.

ALLOXAN

Alloxan is a metabolic by-product created when uric acid is broken down. It is a toxic glucose analogue that selectively destroys pancreatic beta cells which are responsible for producing insulin.

It's a good idea to minimize your intake of purine rich foods that will cause uric acid build-up which in turn will produce trace amounts of alloxan.

Chlorine Dioxide is a whitener used to bleach flour. Trace amounts of this mix with proteins in the flour to form alloxan. Stay away from bleached white flour and anything made from it.

Alloxan is in fact used to deliberately cause a type of diabetes in laboratory animals called alloxan diabetes. It is a potent oxidizing substance and is toxic to the liver kidneys and pancreas.

PANCREATIC CANCER

Diabetics are more at risk of getting pancreatic cancer than most people. Pancreatic cancer is said to be one of the most excruciatingly painful ways to die so avoiding the things that will raise your chances of getting it would be prudent.

There are several risk factors strongly linked to contracting pancreatic cancer. Smoking, obesity, inactivity, diabetes,, high fat diets excessive consumption of red meat ,pork and processed meats are all linked to pancreatic cancer. There are other risk factors but the factors mentioned above in particular are all well within our control.

We can choose to indulge in these things and risk this cancer or we can cut them out of our lives. You can help minimise your risk of contracting this cancer by adding plenty of fresh raw vegetables, rich in folate to your diet and cutting out these risk factors completely.

Cancer cells have insulin receptors on them that allow free glucose to enter so that the cancer cells can grow. Cancer cells do not have the same insulin resistance issues that healthy cells have. We need to minimise both excess glucose and excess insulin in the blood if we are to avoid cancer.

These diseases are all avoided by doing regular exercise and eating a sensible, healthy diet. By reducing stress and not smoking we improve our chances even more.

INSULIN

Insulin is a storage hormone. It is produced in the pancreas to regulate carbohydrate and fat metabolism. It switches on receptors cells in the liver muscles and fat tissue to allow the uptake of glucose from the blood into these cells where it is stored as glycogen. Excess glucose in the blood is toxic so insulin plays a very important role but unfortunately too much insulin in the blood also has serious health implications, i.e. fat storage.

HYPERINSULINEMIA

When the cells of the body become insulin resistant the pancreas responds by producing huge amounts of insulin in an attempt to "force" the glucose into the cells. This results in large amounts of free insulin circulating in the body.

High levels of blood insulin have been linked to sodium retention in the kidneys, obese hypertension and glucose intolerance. It also affects the electrolyte balance within cells by increasing the sodium content and decreasing the potassium content. There is a link between obesity and hyperinsulinemia. What is not known is which one causes the other.

INSULIN RESISTANCE

When there is too much insulin circulating in the blood the receptors that bind to the hormone become increasingly less sensitive to it. The beta cells of the pancreas respond to this by producing even more insulin which contributes even more towards insulin resistance. It puts a massive amount of pressure on the pancreas.

Insulin release is minimised by preventing spikes in blood glucose. You do this by NOT eating high GI/GL foods, by NOT eating high carbohydrate foods and by **eating enough fibre.**

INFLAMMATION

Inflammation is a response by vascular tissues (blood vessels and the circulatory system) to harmful stimuli such as foreign bodies, pathogens, damaged cells, etc. It is very different from infection which is caused by living microorganisms.

Type 2 diabetics appear to have over-active immune responses causing excessive amounts of inflammation-causing toxins in their bodies. **TNF (Tumour Necrosis Factor)** seems to be the prime culprit for causing inflammation. TNF is a pro-inflammatory cytokine created from cells called macrophages. It is a chemical messenger that communicates between cells to provoke an inflammatory response. It is needed to kill cancer cells hence its name **Tumour Necrosis Factor** but too much will actually cause inflammation.

Diabetics are plagued by high levels of inflammation so it is necessary to avoid anything that will stimulate more inflammation. Ripe bananas (the ones with brown spotty skins) contain TNF so if you have trouble with inflammation you may want to avoid eating ripe bananas.

In a healthy person the cells carry distinctive molecules that distinguish them as part of the "self". The immune system does not attack anything with a "self" marker but co-exists in a state of self-tolerance. In an unhealthy individual the immune response cannot distinguish between "self" and "non-self" and the body's own tissues become a target of the immune system.

WHAT CAUSES INFLAMMATION?

There is a theory that Hyperglycaemia (high blood sugar) causes inflammation. Rising blood glucose levels trigger the release of tumour necrosis factor (**TNF** aka **Cachexin** or **Cachectin**) **interleukin-18 (IL-18)** and **C - reactive protein (CRP)**. The presence of these in tests indicates inflammation. They appear to be present solely in a state of hyperglycaemia. A rise in these does not cause a rise in insulin levels.

C-reactive protein (CRP) is a protein found in the blood. It is made by the liver in response to substances released by fat cells. High CRP levels indicate serious infection inflammation and tissue death.

There is a strong connection between the digestive system and the immune system. Diets high in carbohydrates fats refined sugar low protein and low fibre are suspected as the causative agents for inflammation.

Food components like casein and gluten easily set off a cascade of inflammatory hormones like **cytokines, prostaglandins** and **eicosanoids** which cause inflammation. High insulin levels activate enzymes that raise the levels of **arachidonic acid**.

Keeping your blood glucose levels down and stable and avoiding inflammatory foods substances such as gluten or lactose will help to avoid long term health risks and inflammation.

ARACHIDONIC ACID

Arachidonic acid is a polyunsaturated omega-6 essential fatty acid found in animal fats. It is used in the production of hormones and by the immune system. The body needs omega-6 and omega-3 fatty acids to function. The ratio of omega-6 to omega-3 should be 2:1 but in our world today it is more likely to be 20:1. This is due to the way commercial farmers feed our food animals and the use of cooking oils.

Omega-6 fatty acid is vital to the healthy functioning of our bodies but too much will actually stimulate the production of pro-inflammatory prostaglandins thromxanes, lipoxins and leukotrienes. These are collectively known as eicosanoids and are metabolites created from any excess arachidonic acid known as free arachidonic acid. There is a connection between arachidonic acid and diseases such as heart disease, asthma, psoriasis and arthritis.

Arachidonic acid is well documented as a being involved in immunosuppression, thrombosis and inflammation and is well known as a potent platelet aggregator i.e. it is really good at forming blood clots. This is not a good thing if you are having heart or circulation problems since it raises your risk of coronary artery disease, heart attack and stroke. The labels on the "healthy" cooking oils did not warn us about that.

By removing all the causes of inflammation we can move forward in our journey towards a diabetes-free life.

Research done at UCLA has shown that **GABA (Gamma-Amino butyric acid)** may be useful in suppressing these inflammatory immune responses.[7]

Chronic or silent inflammation is implicated as a cause for many illnesses. Too many omega-6 fats and not enough omega-3 fats in our diets cause an imbalance. The omega-6 fats use up all the conversion enzymes leaving nothing for the omega-3 fats (the little we do consume) and cause the production of inflammatory compounds. Because the omega-3 fats are not being converted we do not get any anti-inflammatory benefits from them.

White blood cells are released in a response to inflammation. Too many white blood cells will eventually attack the organs blood vessels and tissues of the body. All of this happens because of too much omega 6 fat and not enough omega-3 fat.

Arachidonic acid is found in commercially farmed duck, chicken, egg yolks, dairy, beef, pork, lamb and fish such as farmed salmon. Ocean caught fish appear to have arachidonic acid content too so this is not an excuse to eat as much fish as you like. Tilapia, catfish, yellowtail and mackerel have higher amounts than other fish.

Organically raised animals tend to have lower amounts of omega-6s and higher amounts of omega-3s, yet another reason to shop organic. Try to cut your animal protein intake down to as little as possible if you do not want to go vegetarian.

It must be said that arachidonic acid is found in greater amounts in the fats of animals so choose the leanest cuts of organic meats if you are going to eat meat. Trim off any visible fat you find.

Food allergies, diet, lifestyle, bacterial imbalance in the intestines, stress and environmental toxicity are all connected to inflammation. What few realise is the connection between inflammation and many diseases like cancer, Alzheimer's, autism, heart disease, depression, dementia and of course diabetes. While taking anti-inflammatory drugs may help in the short term, they are not a long term solution.

Diet, exercise, stress reduction and supplementation with a few selected dietary supplements are all proven long term solutions to reducing inflammation.

Choosing to eat foods that do not stimulate inflammatory responses from the immune system is a good place to start before considering drugs. Fresh, raw vegetables and leafy greens need to be added in abundance to our diets.

Foods like garlic, chilli, ginger, turmeric and berries are all potent anti-inflammatory foods that we should include in greater quantities to our diet. Supplementing with probiotics, cayenne pepper, vitamin D, fish oil and a good quality multivitamin will help to reduce or even stop inflammation.

INFLAMMATORY FOODS

We need a balanced fat intake but also use significantly less fat in total. All fats in excess will have negative consequences but so too will not having any fats at all.

You can be 'skinny" and also have high cholesterol problems. You can also be "skinny" and be diabetic. Being apparently healthy on the outside does not prevent disease from affecting you on the inside. If you are eating unhealthy fats and starches even in smaller amounts you are at risk! How so? By eating foods that promote inflammation!

Canned processed and preserved goods are also high in fats (saturated polyunsaturated and trans-fats), preservatives and sodium. These products are tasty and cheap convenience foods. By trying to save time effort and money we are in fact depriving ourselves of our health. In the long term it costs us in huge medical bills and a shorter lifespan.

The body has fuel resources that it uses in order of preference form quick release to slow release. If you eat enough fast release carbohydrates to meet your energy needs the body will store the slow release energy sources for later. So if you eat plenty fast release carbohydrates and foods high in trans-fats and saturated fats then your body will burn the fast release carbohydrates first and store the fats for later. The problem is that we do not stop eating fast release carbohydrates or high fat foods for long enough to burn them all up. Continuously high blood glucose levels will cause inflammation.

We complicate matters with the addition of high amounts of fructose which is processed by the liver and causes fat to be stored in the liver. 30% of all fructose will be turned into fat regardless of how much or how little of it you eat.

Excess protein consumed will also be converted into uric acid and free amino acids all of which contribute towards inflammation. Food allergies to things such as gluten and lactose have varied levels and many of us do not know we are allergic to them.

If you are eating garbage then garbage is being processed and you start seeing more signs of inflammation by the presence of C-reactive proteins in blood tests. This is caused by the production of toxic metabolites created by eating too much of the wrong types of foods and foods that have little or no active enzymes left in them.

Obesity appears to be a major contributor towards getting diabetes. As fat cells expand they become starved of oxygen and start dying. The cellular death brings the immune response into action!

A gene called 12/15-lipoxygenase (12/15 LO) causes the production of an enzyme that activates white blood cells in the pancreas. The gene is present in the insulin-producing cells in the pancreas and when activated causes these cells to malfunction. A malfunctioning pancreas is a good sign that things have gone horribly wrong somewhere.

SUGAR AND DOPAMINE

The Dopamine Receptor DRD2 plays an important role in diabetes. If you have fewer DRD2 receptors you are more likely to have some sort of addiction problem. It could be drugs alcohol tobacco gambling sex and yes sugar. Researchers also found that diabetics tend to be more likely to have fewer DRD2 receptors.

Sugar affects the dopamine receptors in the rewards centre of the brain in much the same way that heroin or morphine does. It also down regulates them after they have been activated so the next time you need more sugar for the same hit in the same manner as for hard drugs. The more sugar you eat the more you need the next time. You are addicted to sugar and you do not know it!

Having fewer DRD2 receptors is associated with insufficient brain reward meaning you need more of something for less of a "fix'. Overeating and eating the wrong types of foods will be that "fix". It is very convenient then that sugar is so addictive and will easily provide the sought after "hit" or "fix".

The good news is that a low GI high fibre diet can help rectify this with a reduction in blood pressure and body weight as results.[8]

You are what you eat as the saying goes. This is especially true in diabetes. The type of food you eat will determine which genes are activated.

You are going to experience similar withdrawal symptoms to those experienced by drug addicts. These will include headaches mood swings. Get off the sugar(s) now! Cold turkey!

TYPES OF BODYFAT

INTRA MUSCULAR LIPDS (IMCL): is fat stored between muscle fibres like the marbling on a steak. It is thought to be the cause of insulin resistances but recent research suggests IMCL metabolites like diacylglycerol and ceramide are responsible. An increase in adipose (fat) tissue correlates with an increase in IMCL.

LIPID DROPLETS: Also known as intramyocellular lipids, this is fat stored within a cell (in the form of triacylglcerol) for energy. Too much of this within a cell leads to the cell being insulin resistant and not allowing glucose to enter. Glucose is the primary cellular energy source with lipid droplets being used as stored energy. It is one of the reasons a low fat low carbohydrate diet is recommended for diabetics.

There are 2 types of adipose tissue: brown adipose tissue (BAT) and white adipose tissue (WAT). Brown adipose tissue burns fat and white adipose tissue stores fat.

WHITE ADIPOSE TISSUE (WAT)

This fat makes up between 20-25% total bodyweight. WAT cells contain single large fat droplets. WAT has receptors for insulin growth hormones norepinephrine and glucocorticoids. It has 3 functions: insulation cushioning and energy.

White adipose tissue is stored energy. When the pancreas releases insulin the WAT cells cause a dephosphorylation cascade that causes the inactivation of lipase (the fat digesting enzyme).

Conversely when Glucagon is released by the pancreas it re-activates lipase receptors in WAT cells that cause the breakdown of stored fat into fatty acids. The fatty acids are then used as a fuel source by skeletal muscle and cardiac muscle.

WAT tissue functions like an endocrine gland. When it sits around the abdomen it stimulates the release of hormones like adiponectins, resistin and TNF alpha which increase the risk of diabetes and heart disease.

WAT has its uses such as thermal insulation and protecting the internal organs but too much of it is a visible sign of obesity and will also choke or suffocate the organs it is trying to protect.

BROWN ADIPOSE TISSUE (BAT) [9]

This body fat contains numerous smaller fat drops unlike WAT. It is found in greater quantities in infants but is also found in small amounts in adults. Statistics vary as to what percentages of BAT adults actually still have.

In adults it tends to be found in the upper chest and neck around organs with high metabolic activity like the adrenals as well as the liver and kidneys. The iron content of BAT is what makes it brown.

There are more capillaries in BAT than WAT and therefore it has a greater need for oxygen. BAT takes calories from normal fat and uses them as fuel. It is very efficient at using energy. 50g of BAT can burn up to 20% of your daily caloric intake. Its function is to transfer energy from food into heat (taking a cold shower will actually burn fat).[10]BAT is important in weight loss and glucose uptake.[11]

One of BATs functions in adults is thermogenesis (heat generation) which it does by burning WAT. One of the ways it does this is through the protein Thermogenin which is found in the mitochondria of BAT. Thermogenin (found in wakame seaweed) stimulates BAT into burning off WAT tissue.

Studies have suggested that having more BAT may prevent obesity and diabetes suggesting that we need to have more BAT than WAT to be healthy. The polypeptide hormone **Irisin** is needed to ensure that this happens. Irisin is activated through physical exercise and switches on genes that turn WAT into BAT and also improves glucose tolerance. Irisin should be available soon as a weight loss supplement.

Regular exercise increases Irisin levels in the body. When your total body energy expenditure increases your insulin resistance is reduced. Regular vigorous exercise will result in significant improvements in metabolic functions and reduction of inflammation. [12]

BAT is activated by cold so take an ice bath a cold shower and use an icepack on the back of the neck or on your chest or drink ice-water. By activating your BAT you will be burning off WAT essentially losing weight by doing very little at all.

As you age your BAT levels drop but it is possible to keep them activated by ensuring your adrenals and thyroid are

healthy as both play an important role in how BAT is activated.

GLUCAGON

Glucagon is a peptide hormone secreted by the pancreas to raise blood glucose levels. It has the opposite effect to insulin. It tells the liver to convert
stored glycogen to glucose.

Epinephrine (adrenaline) stimulates the release of
glucagon, so remember to avoid stress at all costs if
you do not want high blood glucose levels.

THE SOMOGYI EFFECT

If you wake in the mornings and test your blood glucose
levels to find them high chances are you have experienced
the Somogyi Rebound Effect also known as **rebound hyperglycemia**. You may test your glucose levels before bed
and find them acceptable only wake up and find the level
has risen.

This happens when, during the night, your blood glucose
levels drop dangerously low (hypoglycaemia) and your
body responds by releasing stress hormones like epinephrine (adrenaline) and cortisol and the endocrine hormone
glucagon.

Glucagon causes the liver to release stored glucose to raise the blood glucose levels to compensate and the stress hormones cause insulin resistance which keeps the glucose levels elevated. You may find yourself waking at night sweating and with rapid heart rate which is a side effect of stress hormones.

The Somogyi Effect is thought to be brought on by too much insulin or too strong a dose of metformin which causes hypoglycemia. The body reacts to this by producing more glucose to bring it back into balance. This is complicated by insulin resistance which leads to hyperglycemia.

THE DAWN EFFECT

The Dawn effect is similar but different from the Somogyi effect in that it involves elevated blood glucose levels but these are not associated with nocturnal Hypoglycaemia.

It is believed to be a reaction to the natural release of growth hormones cortisol, epinephrine (adrenaline) and glucagon during the night. There is also the possibility that it is caused by eating carbohydrates at bedtime so it is best to avoid eating anything at least 4 hours before going to sleep.

During sleep the body releases hormones to repair cell damage. These hormones are responsible for raising the blood glucose level. This is again complicated by insulin resistance leading to hyperglycemia.

In either case the results are the same i.e. high blood glucose levels on waking. If you are testing regularly and discover this to be the case you need to tell your doctor about it in order to adjust medication or to analyse what your night time eating patterns are. Eating late at night before going to sleep will negatively affect your blood glucose levels.

The Somogyi Effect and The Dawn Phenomenon are both linked to hormonal imbalances and medication irregularities. Either too much or too little medication is being used. Diet and exercise with the intention of coming off all medications are the only ways to solve these issues.

Have your hormone levels and medication levels checked so that adjustments can be made.

DIABETES: YOU AND YOUR DOCTOR

Whenever a doctor cannot do good he must be kept from doing harm.
-Hippocrates

MEDICALLY TREATING DIABETES

We do not treat diabetes we medicate the symptoms. We use medications to treat the many complications and symptoms of diabetes but we never really get to the root cause of the problem. We use drugs that cause secondary issues to the diseases that they are trying to treat.

METFORMIN (Glucophage): is a biguanide drug that decreases the liver's production of glucose and increases insulin sensitivity in muscles so that they take in more glucose. Metformin also does not cause weight gain and may in fact help with weight loss. Sounds good so far?

The side effects for Metformin are lactic acidosis, gastrointestinal upset, diarrhoea, cramps, nausea, vomiting, blocks the absorption of Vitamins B9 (folic acid) and B12 (cobalamin) raises the blood levels of homocysteine. What does this mean?

Lactic acidosis occurs when there is impaired cellular respiration (the cells are not getting enough oxygen) and they are forced to metabolise glucose anaerobically (without oxygen), causing low ph levels and lactate formation. It is a potentially fatal condition. Metformin is processed by the kidneys and this puts them under more stress if you already suffer from a kidney disease or eat a lot of animal protein.

Metformin blocks Vitamins B9 and B12 which causes homocysteine levels to rise. High levels of Homocysteine are linked to Alzheimer's disease, heart Attack and Stroke.

Supplementing with B Vitamins 9 12 and folic acid help to reduce the blood levels of homocysteine.

STATIN DRUGS: statin drugs do have many good plus points such as lowering CRP levels but they also have negative side effects. They deplete the body of **Co-enzyme Q10 (CoQ10)** which increases the risk of heart disease. They are also linked to muscle pain, fatigue, memory loss and liver toxicity, amongst others.

All the medications used to treat diabetes have side-effects. Your doctor should have explained this to you when they were first prescribed for you. You should also have had the long term effects explained to you. In my personal case these were waved aside as being of less importance than the long term outlook for what diabetes had in store for me!

I became resolved to find a solution despite my doctor's warning that the illness would get progressively worse and that there was no cure.[1] The complicated nature of this disease seems to demand an equally complicated cure!

"Extreme remedies are very appropriate for extreme diseases."

— Hippocrates

---

[1] Medical opinions vary as to whether diabetes can be reversed or not. It can! I had many conflicting opinions from medical professionals on this matter. Find a doctor with a positive disposition.

Diet exercise and weight loss all have an important part to play in beating diabetes. It just requires the right combination of all of them together. There are several celebrities who have reversed their diseases among them Drew Carey, Halle Berry, DeWayne McCulley and Mike Adams. They have all had more than their fair share of commentary opinion and scepticism levelled at them. Actress Halle Berry is reported to have "downgraded" her type 1 diabetes to type 2 diabetes by following a strict diet and exercising.

In my own experience I have had one set of medical professionals say that I would be on medication for the rest of my life and that the disease would get progressively worse and another tell me that if I continued with my diet and exercise I would be off medication in six months! Which one of these medical professionals should I choose to believe?

The fact of the matter is that type 2 diabetes is a metabolic disorder caused by poor diet and lack of exercise and not a random biological occurrence nor is it an hereditary genetic flaw. Over time with the correct nutrition and exercise the body can reboot itself back to healthy.

This has been done before and you can do it too. You just need the determination and willpower to do it. You will need a lot of both!

We should rather focus on the positive and trust in the body's power to heal when provided with the right building materials. You wouldn't build your own home with substandard materials would you? So why do the same with your body? You only get one of those to live in!

Medicating diabetes is the same as putting a Band-Aid over a bullet wound. It will not solve the problem merely disguise it. Blood sugar medications are used to physically force the glucose into the cells. The actual cause of the insulin resistance behind the problem is never addressed.

If you refuse to make lifestyle changes then you should continue to take your medications. This will make your life a little bit easier for the limited amount of time that you have left.

MEDICAL TESTING

There are several tests that you will need to do for the rest of your life. These tests are done to keep an eye on your condition to see if you are getting better or worse.

If you only use medication chances are that it will keep getting progressively worse as time goes by. You may start with 3-4 medications now and find that several years down the road you are taking between 16 and 24 different medications to treat a host of different metabolic failings.

If you follow a good diet and exercise regimen you will see improvements and a reduction in your medication. Depending on your willpower and determination you will come off all medications completely and with time your test results might even be in the normal ranges.

These are a few of the tests that your doctor will or should have done for you on a regular basis:

HbA1C:

Red blood cells are made from haemoglobin. Glucose sticks to red blood cells and creates a glycosylated haemoglobin molecule called HbA1c. The more blood glucose you have the more HbA1c you will have.

Red blood cells live for 8-12 weeks before being replaced and for this reason this test is only done every 3-6 months. It is done to see how well you are managing your blood glucose levels over time.

Blood glucose levels fluctuate very minute of every hour of every day in both non-diabetics and diabetics so this test is done to check the long term blood glucose values. If your HbA1c readings are getting worse then your diabetes is getting worse.

If your HbA1c readings are returning to normal levels then you are getting better. This needs to be done without the use of drugs to be considered a cure and it will also take a few years of diligent diet and exercise.

 Getting your blood sugar down to normal levels is a quick patch-up job; the true cure lies in normal HbA1c levels.

As I write this my test results sit next to me on the desk. My HbA1c level is 36 mmol /mol without the use of any medication. I am within the normal range.

Below is a chart of HbA1c values to use as a reference for when you get your HbA1c levels checked. These values may differ slightly from one country to the next.

	DIABETES	PREDIABETES	NORMAL
PERCENTAGE	6.5 % or more	5.8% - 6.4%	4% - 5.7%
Mmol/mol	48	40 - 47	20 - 39
Mg/dl	140	120 – 137	68 - 117

FRUCTOSAMINE TEST: the Fructosamine test is similar to the HbA1C test. It tests the levels of Glycated Serum Protein (GSP) or Glycated Albumin in the blood. It is a done to monitor changes in diabetic medication over a 2-3 week period rather than a 3 monthly period. It is a good indicator of improvements or setbacks in the short term.

THYROID FUNCTION TEST: This test is done to check your Thyroid Stimulating Hormone (TSH) levels. Hypothyroidism is a potential issue in diabetes. If your thyroid is underactive you are at risk of weight gain and heart disease.

LIPID TEST: This test will check your cholesterol and triglyceride levels. High triglyceride levels are an indication of diabetes, alcoholism, hypothyroidism and obesity.

If your triglycerides are high then you are doing something wrong either too high a fat intake or too high a simple carbohydrate intake.

TRIGYLCERIDES

Triglycerides are the chemical forms of animal and vegetable fats. Three molecules of essential fatty acids combine with glycerol (glycerin) to make a triglyceride.

Triglycerides are created through the intake of fats and carbohydrates. Calories from foods like carbohydrates that are not used for energy immediately are converted to triglycerides and stored in fat cells. Triglycerides are essentially storage lipids (fats).

When the body needs energy but there is no food source for this hormones trigger the release of triglycerides from the fat cells to be used as energy. Glucose is the preferred fuel for most cells but when stored as glycogen in the liver and muscles it takes up space. Triglycerides are a more compact energy source and better for long-term storage than glucose.

If you are overweight, sedentary, smoke, drink too much alcohol and eat a high carbohydrate diet chances are you will have high triglyceride and total cholesterol levels.

If you consistently eat more calories than you burn up you end up with hypertriglyceridemia (high blood levels of fat). This is one of the reasons a low fat calorie restricted diet and exercise is advised for reversing diabetes.

You need to stop eating foods that encourage the storing of energy and burn off any stored energy. This means that the origin of the calories must be scrutinised since calories are NOT all equal.

Alcohol, sugar, fructose and starchy carbohydrates will increase your triglyceride levels. Omega 3 oils and aerobic exercise alongside a low carb diet will help to lower your triglycerides.

RENAL FUNCTION TEST: This test is done to check on the health of your kidneys. It checks the levels of sodium and potassium (electrolytes) as well as Creatinine and uric acid levels. Too much Uric acid will cause gout arthritis and kidney stones. The electrolyte levels will indicate possible dehydration which increases the risk of uric acid build-up.

LIVER FUNCTION TEST: This test is done to check if the liver is working normally by testing the levels of various enzymes in the blood. Liver disease produces very mild symptoms which are easily overlooked until it is too late to do anything about.

CHOLESTEROL: everybody gets their cholesterol checked at some point but what do we actually know about this stuff?

Cholesterol is a white waxy lipid (water insoluble) substance found inside the cell membranes and acts as a kind of glue to hold those membranes together. All animal proteins contain cholesterol even fish and seafood. It is an essential structural building block of cell membranes.

80-90% of the cholesterol in your body is made by the body itself in the liver. This means that 10-20% of the total cholesterol in your body will come from your diet. It is possible to be a vegan and have high cholesterol if your diet includes polyunsaturated fats and is high in carbohydrates (sugar, fructose, grains and starchy carbohydrates).

Similarly even if you eat no fat at all you can still get fat if you consume large amounts of fructose since at least 30% of all fructose ingested will end up as fat. A low fat diet is NOT a low fat diet if it contains too many refined carbohydrates or fructose.

Cholesterol is an essential building block of many hormones. It is used to make stress and sex hormones like testosterone, oestrogen, progesterone, aldosterone and cortisol. The liver turns cholesterol into bile salts necessary for the absorption of fats and fat soluble vitamins like Vitamin A D and K. under the influence of UVB rays the skin turns cholesterol into vitamin D.

It is needed for intracellular transport nerve conduction cell signalling and repairing damage to arteries.

Although cholesterol is important, too much of it in our bodies is very unhealthy for us. The liver produces about 1000mg per day and our average daily consumption is about 150-250mg on top of that. The liver sends cholesterol into the bloodstream so that your cells can make use of it.

Cholesterol cannot travel through the bloodstream by itself so it has to combine with certain proteins which act as transport vehicles for it. Together they are called a lipoprotein. This is how we get high-density lipoproteins (**HDL**) (good) and low-density lipoproteins (**LDL**) (bad). There is a third type of cholesterol called very low density lipoprotein (**VLDL**) (very bad) and this is by far the most dangerous type.

The term cholesterol is a bit misleading since cholesterol only a component of lipoproteins.

In order for cholesterol to move around the body it needs to bind with a protein (lipid + .protein makes a lipoprotein). There are two important forms of lipoprotein: HDL and LDL cholesterol.

LDL (known as bad cholesterol) contains more cholesterol than protein and is heavier and slower than HDL. LDL is transported from the liver to where it is needed. Cells have special receptors that attach to LDL as it passes by. Soluble fibre such as that found in oats, barley, beans and lentils will help to lower LDL. Weight loss diet exercise and quitting smoking will help to reduce LDL cholesterol.

HDL (known as good cholesterol) contains more protein than cholesterol and moves faster than LDL through the body. It transports cholesterol back to the liver to be converted to bile acids. Eating olives, olive oil, nuts and seeds will help to raise HDL levels and lower LDL levels walnuts flaxseeds and fatty fish contain omega-3 fatty acids that will also help to raise HDL levels. .

What really matters is the ratio of LDL to HDL cholesterol. This is a good indication of the risk of heart attack or heart disease. A ratio of 3.3 or 4.4 LDL to HDL is considered a low risk of heart but a ratio of 7.1 or higher of LDL to HDL is considered a high risk.

Research has shown that a modest intake of alcohol around 1 drink per day can lower LDL cholesterol and raise HDL cholesterol. It is also believed to reduce blood clotting and insulin resistance and lower levels of C-reactive protein which is a marker for heart disease. Several studies have shown evidence to suggest that people who drink moderate amounts of alcohol (1 drink per day) have lower rates of heart disease. Red wine is of particular interest as it contains resveratrol. Drinking too much alcohol actually raises the risk of heart disease.

Too much cholesterol in the blood can result in plaques forming on artery walls. This is called atherosclerosis. Plaques can crack or rupture which causes the blood in that area to clot which if it happens in the heart becomes a heart attack. If it happens in the brain it becomes a stroke. It can also cause significant damage to other areas of the body.

LDL is the bad stuff that is most likely to clog arteries and HDL is the good stuff that moves from the blood vessels back to the liver for processing and removal from the body.

Atherosclerosis is an inflammatory process caused by a diet that is too high in refined and starchy carbohydrates and omega-6 vegetable oils alongside vitamin and mineral deficiencies bacterial infections and chronic stress. Cholesterol is used to repair the damage but if the damage is continuous and needs to be constantly repaired then the repair work can become the damage.

Cholesterol is recycled. The liver excretes cholesterol via the bile into the digestive tract. 50% of this cholesterol is then re-absorbed back into the bloodstream via the small bowel. The more animal protein you eat the more cholesterol you will have. Almonds olive oil blueberries avocado tomato oatmeal and cocoa (not chocolate bars) have all been reported as beneficial dietary inclusions that will lower cholesterol.

Cholesterol is a vitally important component in cell membranes nerve and brain tissue. Studies have shown that older patients with higher cholesterol levels live longer than patients of the same age with lower cholesterol levels. If you are healthy you can have high cholesterol levels without incidents but if you have chronic inflammation high cholesterol levels can be life threatening.

New research is suggesting that removing refined carbohydrates from your diet and a modest intake of saturated and monounsaturated fats are the key to keeping cholesterol in check.

Taking a low dose aspirin daily will help to prevent plaque build-up in the artery walls.

NOTES

QUICKSTART GUIDE

"Always do what you are afraid to do."

– Ralph Waldo Emerson

STOP DOING THAT RIGHT NOW

Here's a list of a few things you need to stop doing immediately.

1. Stop eating refined **starchy carbohydrates** like bread, pasta, cereals, white rice and potatoes. Anything white and starchy should be avoided.

2. Stop eating **sugar** or anything sweet including fruit.

3. Stop drinking fruit juice or anything containing **fructose.**

4. Stop using **Caffeine**

5. Stop Eating **Dairy** products including goat or sheep.

6. Stop consuming **processed** foods, canned meals[2] processed meat and related products instant foods take-out or convenience foods. Eat raw unprocessed foods as much as possible.

7. Stop eating fried foods, high fat foods and cooking **oils/fats.**

8. Adjust your **protein** intake.

9. Stop using **nicotine.**

10. Stop using **alcohol**. Alcohol provides empty, liquid calories and raises cholesterol and uric acid levels.

11. Stop Using **Artificial Sweeteners**[3]

12. Stop **stressing.**

---

[2] By canned meals I mean seasoned, flavoured products which are high in salt and fat. Read the labels carefully.

[3] Aspartame produces formaldehyde as a by-product when metabolised. Natural sweeteners like Xylitol and Stevia are acceptable. Several studies have shown that some artificial sweeteners will stimulate carbohydrate cravings and fat storage.

1: STARCHY CARBOHYDRATES ¹³

Carbohydrates come exclusively from plants in the form of either starches or sugars. These are refined and processed to create alcohol or crystalline sucrose or fructose or made into bread or pasta. You can also drink carbohydrates in the form of a can of beer or a glass of juice. Carbohydrates that have been stripped of all there fibre will rapidly raise blood glucose levels.

There are two types of carbohydrate:

SIMPLE CARBOHYDRATES: examples of these are sugar, fruit juice, white bread, cakes etc. these are foods or ingredients that rapidly raise blood sugar levels and have little to no fibre content at all.

COMPLEX CARBOHYDRATES: examples of these are whole fruits and vegetables, wholegrains, pulses and legumes. These will lots of fibre to slow down the absorption of glucose and maintain steady blood glucose levels.

Wheat flour and any products made from it such as bread, pasta, biscuits, crackers, pastries, cakes, etc. are carbohydrates. White or refined rice and anything made from rice flour, crisps, potatoes and anything made from potato flour, french fries, corn and corn products (high fructose corn syrup is made from corn!) sugar, soda (diet and regular), cakes, pies, pastries, cookies, bread crumbs, cereals, crackers, pasta, bread, processed honey (usually cut with sugar to extend it), snack foods (even "healthy "ones), jellies, jams, donuts etc. are all carbohydrates to be avoided.

White flour contains trace amounts of Alloxan. It is a by-product of the bleaching process for wheat flour. Chlorine Dioxide used to bleach flour binds with protein to form alloxan. It is used in laboratories to artificially create a type of insulin-dependent diabetes (alloxan diabetes) in lab animals. Vitamin E supplementation is said to be used to undo this type of diabetes in lab animals. Brown flour is simply white flour with added wheat bran so don't be fooled into thinking it's "healthy".

Proteins and fats do not have a dramatic effect on blood sugar levels starchy carbohydrates do!

Fats will raise blood glucose in 6-8 hours after a meal; proteins will raise blood glucose in 3-4 hours after a meal. Carbohydrates show up as blood glucose in half an hour to an hour after a meal.

Refined starchy carbohydrates are more troublesome as they release a huge hit of blood glucose without the benefit of fibre to slow down the conversion from starch to glucose.

We need to eliminate them from our diets in order to minimise the spike in blood sugar that they cause. We rely too much on starchy carbs filling us up and we lose out on quality nutrition from other foods.

Fibre plays an important role in slowing down the rate at which food is broken down into glucose and most refined carbohydrates are lacking in fibre.

Carbohydrates are converted to glucose. Insulin decides what will happen to both glucose and dietary fat whether they will be used as fuel or stored as fat. Having too much fat alongside too much refined carbohydrate in your diet will raise both your cholesterol and blood glucose levels.

If there is too much blood glucose available it will cause fat to be stored. Some of the glucose will also be stored as fat. You now have fat from two sources being stored.

Saturated fats are healthy in small amounts but refined simple carbohydrates in the amounts that we are currently consuming are not. We need to eliminate the refined carbohydrates and be more sensible about our fat intake.

Sugar is a refined carbohydrate and is found in almost everything we consume these days. You will need to start reading labels on everything you purchase. Sugar is simply empty calories with no nutritional benefit whatsoever.

Do not be fooled by sugar substitutes and artificial sweeteners. Some of them are excitotoxic and destroy nerve cells and others will cause gastric distress in sufficient quantities. Just quit cold turkey and do not try to fool yourself or your body with additional poisons.

2: SUGAR

Sugar is a concentrated source of calories. It will raise your blood glucose levels immediately. The worst aspect about sugar metabolism is that 50% of all sugar ingested will be turned into fructose which goes straight to the liver.

We have all been told to stay away from sugar, so, enough said!

3: FRUCTOSE AND FRUIT

Try to minimise your fruit intake or completely eliminate fruit and particularly fruit juice from your diet .Why? Fruit is healthy right?

Fruit and anything with sugar in it will be high in fructose[14]. Why is this bad? Fructose is converted to Glycerol Phosphate which plays an important part in binding free fatty acids to form triglycerides (test subjects fed large amounts of fructose were discovered to have high triglycerides.) Therefore fructose equals triglycerides.

The liver is responsible for filtering out toxins and 100% of fructose consumed gets processed by it and 30% of all fructose will be turned into fat. This alone should raise warning flags. The body does not know what to do with fructose except store it as fat in the form of triglycerides.

Fructose metabolism causes the production of Xylulose-5-P which creates more fat storage enzymes leading to the production of VLDL (very low density lipoprotein) which contains the highest amounts of triglycerides of all the cholesterols i.e. you have just dramatically increased your risk of heart disease.

VLDL is the most dangerous form of cholesterol. It is made of small dense particles that get under the endothelial plates causing plaque formation. When getting your blood tested you should be looking for **low** levels of **triglycerides** and **high** levels of **HDL** as this is a good sign.

High triglycerides and **low HDL** levels are going to lead you to a heart attack. This is a bad thing.

Fructose is also linked to high blood pressure and insulin resistance.[15]

A waste product of fructose metabolism is uric acid. Uric acid causes the endothelial cells (arterial cells) to reduce production of nitric oxide. Nitric oxide keeps the arteries dilated (open). If there is not enough nitric oxide available then the arteries are constricted (closed) which means high blood pressure and increased risk of heart attack and stroke and reduced blood flow to the brain.[16]

If you cannot live without fruit then try to minimise the amount you consume and focus only on low GL fruits like berries grapefruit apples peaches apricots etc. Do searches on which fruits have a low GI/GL and stick to them exclusively if you absolutely must have fruit.

Do not drink fruit juice. It is a concentrated source of fructose. If you must have fruit juice then drink grapefruit juice if you are allowed to (some medications are enhanced by grapefruit juice) or dilute your fruit juice 50/50 with filtered water and again limit the amount you drink.

Fruit juice specifically the fructose in it does not stimulate a Ghrelin response meaning you do not feel full no matter how much you drink. Because fructose does not stimulate insulin or leptin production it can easily lead to overeating. You still feel hungry afterwards so you keep on eating.

The fibre in fruit slows down the absorption of fructose in a strange case of the poison being administered with the remedy as Professor Robert H. Lustig is quoted as saying "when God made the poison He packaged it with the antidote: fibre". This is not the case with fruit juice which is basically concentrated fruit with no fibre to slow down the absorption of the fructose.

In the past fruit was seasonal. Our ancestors ate fruit straight from the tree and dried the fruit the excess fruit for the lean months ahead. The fructose that would become stored fat would serve them well over the cold lean winter months.

Fruit is no longer seasonal. We have access to fruit 24/7/365. We have fruit juice that our ancestors did not have. We have an endless supply of concentrated poison now and none of the antidote.

In his book "the 4 hour body" Timothy Ferriss notes that a diet with elevated fructose content will raise cholesterol albumin and iron levels dramatically. Albumin binds to testosterone making it less available and excessive levels of iron in the system can be toxic.

Fructose Metabolism
Sugar (sucrose) is made up of 50% glucose and 50% fructose which are found in abundance in fruit and fruit juice.

All fructose ingested goes straight to the liver to be processed. A by-product of fructose metabolism is uric acid. Uric acid causes the endothelial cells to reduce their production of nitric oxide. Nitric oxide keeps arteries dilated. Less nitric oxide means constricted arteries which mean higher blood pressure i.e. Fructose raises blood pressure. There is a connection between high uric acid levels and hypertension.[17]

Other by-products are xylulose-5-P which causes an increase in fat storage enzymes and pyruvate which becomes Acetyl-CoA which becomes citrate.

The fat storing enzymes work with the citrate to form VLDL (very low density lipoprotein) the most dangerous form of cholesterol as well as fat. Fructose is the biggest generator of VLDL.

There is also the production of lipid droplets which settle in the liver causing a fatty liver and FFA (free fatty acids) which settle in the muscle tissue (as intramuscular lipids IMCL) causing muscular insulin resistance. More insulin in the blood correlates with more fat storage.

Mitogen-activated protein kinase 8 (also known as JNK1 or junk 1) is also formed as a by-product of fructose metabolism. This enzyme is produced in the liver and causes the liver's insulin receptors to become insulin resistant. This raises the insulin levels in the blood. High levels of insulin in the system mask the presence of leptin. Leptin is the hormone responsible for telling the brain that you are full so you can stop eating. If your brain does not recognize the presence of leptin it assumes that you have not eaten enough so you stay hungry and keep on eating.

There is not one single biological process in the human body that requires fructose or sucrose. They will be turned into stored energy! Any energy that we need we get from our food or from stored fat. Dietary intake of fructose and sucrose is equivalent ingesting toxins.
Here are a few points about fructose metabolism:

- **Advanced Glycation End Products (AGE's):** Fructose is 7-10 times more likely to form AGE's (by-products that are linked to aging cardiovascular disease Alzheimer's stroke inflammation wrinkles (damaged collagen) and the cross-linking of proteins that can cause cancer.)

- **Ghrelin dysfunction:** Fructose does not suppress ghrelin (the hunger hormone) so you stay feeling hungry when you eat it.
- **Leptin dysfunction:** Fructose does not stimulate leptin. The satiety hormone that tells you when are full. This leads to overeating.
- **Hypertension:** Fructose makes a waste product that increases uric acid that blocks the enzyme our bodies need to make nitric oxide (NO) which lowers blood pressure and dilates (opens) blood vessels. That translates into high blood pressure.
- **Elevated triglycerides**: fructose raises triglyceride levels
- **Hepatic (liver) insulin resistance**. Fructose can cause liver insulin resistance (and thus making the pancreas work harder) increasing lipid droplet (fat inside the cells) in the liver. It can cause non-alcoholic fatty liver disease (NAFLD).
- **Uric Acid:** production of which leads to gout.
- **Free Fatty Acids (FFA)**: a by-product of fructose metabolism is turned into intramyocellular fat leading to insulin resistance and beta-cell dysfunction.
- **JNK1 (junk 1):** production leads to liver insulin resistance.
- **Novo Lipogenesis:** Fructose increases this process which causes 30% of calories from fructose to turn into fat making a high sugar diet essentially a high fat diet.

CONCLUSION:
STAY THE HELL AWAY FROM FRUCTOSE!

Diabetes high blood pressure heart disease high cholesterol and gout are all linked to fructose. This stuff is poison! It is hepatotoxic!

Fruit juice, honey, rice syrup, agave syrup, maple syrup, and any other "natural" syrup you might find will contain fructose so avoid at all costs. Stevia and luo han guo fruit extract do not contain fructose.

Now that I have bashed the hell out of fruit and fruit juice I need to say that the occasional piece of fruit is acceptable and healthy as long as it is eaten with its natural fibre content in other words as nature intended.

Fruits contain various phytochemicals just like vegetables do and each will have its own purpose and function, like **naringenin** in grapefruit or **bromelain** in pineapple. This needs to be acknowledged, but not indulged in. Fruit is sweet and should be seen as a treat for occasional consumption only.

Educate yourself on the various fruits and what phytochemicals they contain and eat them, whole, for their health properties occasionally. Remember that food is medicine but it can very easily become poison.

AGEs (ADVANCED GLYCATION ENDPRODUCTS)

These are toxic products that result from the process known as Glycation. Glycation is what happens when a sugar molecule bonds with a fat or a protein molecule.

Glycation is an uncontrolled non-enzymatic process that changes the structure and function of proteins within the body.

When a protein molecule and a sugar molecule are cross-linked through Glycation an AGE is created.[18] AGEs are inflammatory compounds that are thought to be one of the leading causes of aging.

There are 2 types of AGEs:

Exogenous or dietary AGEs are formed when sugars are cooked with fats and/or proteins.
Examples of this would be french fries, donuts, fudge, dark coloured soda, barbecued meats and sauces and anything that has been "browned" or "caramelized".

Endogenous Glycation occurs inside the body mainly in the bloodstream. Fructose has ten times the Glycation activity (AGE producing ability) of glucose.

Hyperglycaemia (high blood glucose) increases AGE production beyond normal levels. AGEs are linked to a long list of diseases and conditions notably atherosclerosis heart disease gum disease kidney disease Alzheimer's cancer and eye disease.

Adding sugar to egg whites will increase AGE production by 200 per cent. This means no more meringues or nougat

If AGEs are allowed to continue being formed particularly in the case of diabetics the end result will usually be a kidney transplant or dialysis. A little bit of fructose is not worth all the risks involved. Many sweeteners are fructose derived so be careful with your choices of apparently safe alternatives.

Vegetables should be eaten raw or lightly steamed, never fried. If you eat meat it should be cooked low and slow and never barbecued or fried. Eggs should be boiled poached or steam-fried. Do not use oil to cook protein or sugars with as it will cause the formation of AGEs.

Alpha lipoic acid, aspirin, carnosine, pyridoxamine (vitamin B6,) and resveratrol are used to control and inhibit AGE formation.

4: CAFFEINE [19] [20]

Caffeine stimulates insulin surges. There is data to suggest that excessive use may cause the body to produce trace amounts of Alloxan.

Caffeine appears to exaggerate the level of glucose in the blood when consumed with food.[21] Eating a high GI snack with your coffee (donut croissant muffin etc.) will increase the levels of glucose in your bloodstream by 300% while halving the amount of insulin required regulating it.

Caffeine also raises the levels of **homocysteine C-reactive protein (CRP)** and **tumour necrosis factor (TNF).**Try herbal teas such as redbush (rooibos) or any of the hundreds of other non-caffeine herbal teas instead.

There is hope yet! Try **decaffeinated coffee**. Decaf contains caffeic acid which has shown anti-oxidant and anti-carcinogenic properties. Chlorogenic acid in decaf can reduce the production of glucose by the liver and also lessens the hyperglycaemic peak in the blood after the consumption of sugar.

Coffee beans contain chlorogenic acid to defend against virus's bacteria and fungi which may be of benefit for us. Ferulic acid is an antioxidant which neutralizes free radicals and may prevent oxidative damage caused by exposure to UV light. Ferulic acid also decreases blood glucose levels and reduces the level of cholesterol and triglycerides. Ferulic acid is also a potent anti-inflammatory capable of significantly reducing brain inflammation.

5: DAIRY

Our lactase enzyme the enzyme allowing us to digest dairy products begins to decline as we age leading to numerous health issues best avoided by diabetics.

As you have also read in the beginning of the book there is a connection between insulin producing pancreatic beta-cell damage caused by an immune response to a milk protein that mimics the islet cell protein of the insulin producing cells.

The risks appear to be greater for infants with weak immune systems than for adults but there are risks nevertheless. A compromised immune system may leave the door open for other risks factors to become a reality.

Most of us hardly notice the effects that dairy has on us until we give it up. Only then do we realise the negative health effects.

LACTOSE: lactose is the sugar component found in ALL dairy products. This means that dairy products from sheep, goat, cow and buffalo will **all** contain various amounts of lactose.

Lactose is a disaccharide sugar that is converted into glucose and galactose. Galactose is converted by the liver into glucose when called for.

Lactose will raise your blood glucose levels but this happens gradually as the protein in dairy slows down the digestion of the dairy. This means it will take a little longer to be released as blood glucose.

Lactose intolerance is not a modern illness either. Otzi the 5000 year old iceman discovered frozen in the Alps was discovered to carry the genome for lactose intolerance. It is believed that up to 70% of the total world population have some degree of lactose intolerance. Certain populations will have a greater or lesser degree of intolerance than others but you will not know unless you get tested.

Natural live yoghurt does not appear to cause any trouble and due to its live bacterial cultures is actually beneficial to your digestive health. Dairy products from goat or sheep are a healthier alternative if you absolutely must have cheese or dairy products. That being said both goat and sheep dairy products both contain lactose, the sugar component of dairy products. The protein and fat components are different from bovine dairy since they are different animals but if you are lactose intolerant you will not have any luck with sheep or goat dairy products.

Dairy is also a source of saturated fats and cholesterol which leads to intramyocellular lipid build-up a cause of insulin resistance. If you suffer from inflammation you should avoid all dairy products.

Although dairy products are low GI (i.e. they do not spike blood glucose levels) dairy is extremely insulinogenic (it will dramatically spike your insulin levels). This is called hyperinsulinemia and is believed to be one of the causes of hyperglycaemia (diabetes).

If you are insulin resistant, consuming insulinogenic foods will raise your blood insulin levels and increase your insulin resistance. You do not want to spike your insulin levels any more than you want to spike your glucose levels so stay away from dairy.

 The treatment for hyperinsulinemia is the same as for hyperglycaemia in that diet exercise and metformin are common to both. Cinnamon and cinnamon extract has also been used effectively as a treatment for both of these conditions.

Lactose may be one of the issues with dairy, but another issue had recently come to light. That issue is one of addiction. Dairy products contain casein which is a milk protein. Casein contains protein segments called peptides and one of these peptides is called casomorphins.

Casomorphins are opioid peptides, meaning they have an opioid or addictive effect on us. This literally means that ALL dairy products are addictive to some degree.

Dairy also raises IGF-1 (insulin-like growth factor) levels in the human body. What it does is promote growth (like calves or babies), but it also increases the growth of cancer cells

Milk, from any dairy source, is designed to promote the growth and immunity of the infant from whatever species produced that milk. It is not for fully grown adults, or even adolescents, from a different species. Studies have shown that higher IGF-1 levels also correlate with shorter life spans and higher cancer rates.

If you find dairy difficult to give up, now you know why.

6: PROCESSED FOODS

Processed foods are usually high in sodium, trans-fats, preservatives and fillers. They are nutritionally poor high GI / GL and low fibre. Processed foods are designed to have extended shelf life. They are NOT designed to be nutritious. They are designed to taste good so that you buy more. They are designed to sit on a supermarket or cupboard shelf for long periods of time so that they are more profitable.

A product that has an extended shelf life will have preservatives in it. Preservatives are **poisons** that kill or prevent organisms from multiplying. Processed foods will only have the basic nutritional components like protein and energy and possibly added cheap vitamins to create the illusion of nutrition.

Stop eating ALL processed meats (polonies, salami, sausage, ham, bacon etc.) and ready-made ready-to-eat instant anything even if it claims to be low fat or is marketed as healthy. It is not!

These foods have nitrates, nitrites, benzoates and sulphites. These and other preservatives have been linked to many serious health issues such as allergies, asthma, high blood pressure, high cholesterol, kidney failure, liver damage, strokes, heat attacks and cancer. Your food is killing you! When your food has a longer life than you do something is not right.

Processed foods will also have trans-fats and polyunsaturated fats in them. Excessive amounts of these will lead to heart disease and diabetes. These foods have only the basics like fat carbohydrates and proteins left in them. Any other nutritional value will have been stripped during processing. Sodium and sugar are what accounts for the tastiness of processed foods. We need the extra salt and sugar right?

These foods are not designed to be nutritious. They are designed to sit on a shelf for ages and to generate a profit. The cost of all this is your health! Stay away from processed foods as much as possible!

If it's made by man, throw it in the garbage can!

7: FAT: THE GOOD THE BAD AND THE UGLY

Fatty acids are the primary sources of fuel for many tissues. Cells can use either glucose or fatty acids as fuel. Studies have shown that the heart and skeletal muscles can use fatty acids but the brain can only use ketones.

SATURATED FAT: found in animal fats such as organic or raw butter and tropical fats such as coconut oil, cocoa butter and red palm oil. They are typically solid at room temperature.

These are medium chain fatty acids that are easily and quickly used as energy. Saturated fats are needed for energy and hormone production cellular membranes brain function immune system function and organ insulation. Saturated fats are needed for many vitamins and minerals to be utilized. Calcium needs saturated fat to be taken up by the bones.

When saturated fats are eaten without dietary sugars or starches they are converted into ketones with nitrogen and stored as energy (ATP). This keeps glucose levels steady. The body uses ketones for fuel when there is an absence of glucose.

Recent studies have shown that diets with higher saturated fat content seem to have fewer incidences of heart disease and diabetes than would be expected. [22] [23]

Studies have also shown that ethnic populations that change from using saturated fats such as coconut oil to using polyunsaturated fats develop higher risks of cancer hypothyroidism heart disease high cholesterol and diabetes. Coconut oil helps protect against the anti-thyroid effects of too many unsaturated fats.

There is evidence to suggest that saturated fats are not responsible for heart disease and high cholesterol s we have all been lead to believe.[24]

When saturated fat such as organic butter or coconut oil intake is replaced by trans-fats or polyunsaturated fats and refined carbohydrates such as breads pasta rice sugar fructose etc. the risk of heart disease obesity and diabetes dramatically increases.[25]

The Framingham Heart Study started in 1948 and now in its third generation is an on-going research study into the causes behind heart disease. It has been the biggest study ever undertaken to discover the causes behind heart diseases of all kinds.

They have made some surprising discoveries.

Dr. William Castelli ex-director of the Framingham Heart Study is quoted as saying:

"In Framingham Mass. the more saturated fat one ate the more cholesterol one ate the more calories one ate the lower the person's serum cholesterol. The opposite of what... Keys et al would predict...We found that the people who ate the most cholesterol ate the most saturated fat ate the most calories weighed the least and were the most physically active."

Please do not take this as permission to eat whatever you want to now! This statement did not account for diabetics. The people about whom this was said were active healthy people. It turns the healthy fat dogma upside down and it suggests that some saturated fat intake can be healthy.

Medium chain saturated fats are chemically stable meaning they won't turn rancid and oxidize inside the body.

Approximately 7-10% of your total daily calories from saturated fat is considered a healthy amount. This is around 20g in the average healthy adult.

This is not permission to go out and eat junk food to your heart's desire! It means that a small amount of saturated fat from organic sources is natural and beneficial to health. Too much is just as dangerous as too little.

MONOUNSATURATED FATTY ACIDS

(MUFA): olives peanuts hazel nuts avocados. The fatty acids found in monounsaturated fats help with weight loss to lower cholesterol and are brain and heart healthy. They help to control both insulin and blood glucose levels.

Cold pressed extra virgin olive oil and cold pressed virgin avocado oil are the only oils you should consider using and then only in tiny amounts for salad dressings etc. They are not to be used for cooking at all only as dressings on salads. Always buy these oils in a dark glass bottle to minimise the risk of oxidization caused by exposure to light.

POLYUNSATURATED FATTY ACIDS

(PUFA): are found in omega-6 nut and seed oils and omega-3 marine oils such as krill oil and fish oil supplements. These are made from long chain fatty acids that get stored as cholesterol in the blood vessels.

High intake of polyunsaturated oils has been linked to hypothyroidism. It seems as if unsaturated fats have the ability to interfere with thyroid hormone secretion and the way that thyroid hormones function in the body. The more unsaturated the oil is the greater its effect will be on the thyroid. Unsaturated oils affect the secretion of thyroid hormones the transportation of thyroid hormones in the blood and the response of thyroid tissue receptors.

Since the thyroid controls cholesterol levels in the body unsaturated fats may in fact be causing high cholesterol if they are interfering with the thyroid gland. Several studies have shown that diets high in omega-6 polyunsaturated vegetable oils are linked to higher incidences of diabetes and heart disease. A diet high in polyunsaturated fats has also been linked to heart tissue necrosis[26] [27]. This begs the questions of whether or not polyunsaturated oils are really as heart healthy as they are claimed to be.

A diet high in omega-6 polyunsaturated fat will increase the risks of heart disease diabetes high blood pressure hyperinsulinemia insulin resistance and cancer.[28]

These are worst case scenarios in diets where there are very high amounts of PUFA from fried foods etc. we need PUFA to maintain healthy hearts.

Get your PUFA from raw food sources rather than from oils. Polyunsaturated fats are very unstable due to their many bonds (poly) and go rancid quickly. This implies that they oxidize easily inside the body causing oxidative damage. They are easily damaged by normal cooking temperatures which cause toxic and carcinogenic compounds to be formed.

Cooking oils will contain chemicals that prevent the oils from going rancid or may have been processed at extremely high temperatures.

TRANS FATS: are created artificially by partially hydrogenating unsaturated vegetable oils. Margarine and synthetic cheese are examples of Trans -fats.

While both trans-fats and saturated fats will raise LDL (bad) cholesterol levels trans-fats will also strip away HDL (good) cholesterol and raise triglyceride levels. Trans-fats are used extensively in processed foods.

To create trans-fats essentially means taking a good unsaturated fat and turning it into a saturated fat to improve its shelf life and increase its volume. This also means increasing the risk of coronary heart disease for whoever consumes it.

Saturated fats are found in butter, cheese, lard, suet, cream, fatty meat, palm kernel oil cottonseed oil, chocolate and coconut oil.[4] Certain polyunsaturated oils should also be

---

[4] Coconut oil is actually a good saturated fat. It is a medium-chain fatty acid which means it is used immediately as a fuel source and not stored in the body as a reserve like other saturated fats. It is reputed to have anti-fungal, anti-viral and anti-bacterial properties due to the immune boosting medium-chain fatty acids Caproic

avoided. Canola sunflower and corn oil easily become rancid and may lower good HDL cholesterol when they are denatured by high temperatures. They also become potentially carcinogenic.

Hydrogenated oils are made by heating oil at extremely high temperatures with nickel or aluminium and bubbling hydrogen through it for several hours. This creates a trans-fatty acid. It will never spoil or need refrigeration and has an eternal shelf life. Good for profit toxic for you.

These trans-fatty acids disrupt prostaglandins (bio-chemicals) which regulate things like blood pressure kidney and heart function and the immune system. There is also a link between trans-fat consumption and the development of diabetes.

This may be due to insulin resistance caused by intra-myocellular fat production. The body has great difficulty getting rid of trans-fats so it stores them. The cellular mitochondria are unable to digest trans- fats. Stay away from hydrogenated anything!

Much has been said about a calorie being just a calorie but this is simply not true. All fats are worth 9 calories per gram. There is a world of difference between 1 gram of trans-fats and 1 gram of omega 3 fat in terms of their impact on your health. A calorie is not just a calorie.

---

acid, Caprylic acid, Lauric acid and Myristic acid. Only virgin, cold pressed coconut oil should be used.

Watching your caloric intake is important but of greater significance is the origin of those calories. There are good calories and there are bad calories, do not let the science or the food labels fool you.

FAT CONSUMPTION
We need to eat less fat in total but we also need to be realistic about what types of fat we eat. Most of us have been trained to believe that saturated fat is bad and that polyunsaturated fat is good.

That seems like permission to eat as much of the "healthy" fat as we like and completely avoid the "bad" fat. Unfortunately it is not as simple as that.

We need the "bad" as much as we need the "good" fats. New research is proving that too much polyunsaturated fats can have just as negative an impact on heart health as saturated fats. The lines are becoming blurred.

A recent study [29] done to assess the nutritional factors involved in heart disease found some unusual facts.

Diets with a higher consumption of :

Alcohol, Beta-carotene, fibre, fish, marine omega-3 fats, fruit, vegetables, nuts, folate, monounsaturated fats (olive oil), wholegrains and vitamins C and E had significantly reduced risks of heart disease.

114

Polyunsaturated fats did **NOT** offer any additional protection against heart disease.

Diets with a higher consumption of :

Trans-fatty acids (margarine and vegetable shortening) and high GI and high GL foods had a significantly greater risk of developing heart disease.

Saturated fats did **NOT** contribute to a greater risk of heart disease.

This means that some saturated fat is acceptable and that polyunsaturated fat is not the heart friendly miracle we thought it was.
There are a few studies that disprove the popular belief that saturated fats are bad.[30] [31]

It would seem as if small amounts of saturated fats with modest amounts of monounsaturated fats and some marine sourced omega-3 fats would be healthier than low fat or no fats at all.

It would also appear that using "healthy" polyunsaturated fats with starchy carbohydrates will increase the risk of heart disease and diabetes and NOT reduce those risks as we have all been lead to believe.

Our bodies DO can process small amounts of naturally occurring saturated fats. we can process and utilise small amounts of saturated fats. Small amounts, not bottles or tubs of the stuff.

Our bodies do NOT understand how to process vast quantities of healthy" polyunsaturated fats. We need these fats to be healthy, this is true, but NOT in the quantities that we currently consume them in.

 These fats need to come from nuts and seeds in our diets and **not from bottles on supermarket shelves**.

In years past we were told that trans-fats from margarine or vegetable shortening were safe. We now know this to be false deadly in fact. What other un-truths have we been told?

The key to keeping cholesterol in check and minimise the risk of heart disease is to restrict refined carbohydrate intake as much as possible particularly when there is a high intake of polyunsaturated fats.

No more bread pasta rice fries mashed potatoes or sugars and sweet foods with unsaturated fats if you want to keep heart disease and diabetes at bay.

I do realise the contradictions in telling diabetics that saturated fats are now safe to eat and that polyunsaturated fats are now unsafe but the facts have changed and we need to listen to empirical evidence and not the advertisements of the people trying to sell us a product.

Small amounts of medium chain saturated fats(coconut oil) and monounsaturated fats (olive oil) are proving to be of greater benefit to health than trans-fats (margarine and vegetable shortening) and polyunsaturated fats (canola sunflower safflower sesame corn peanut and soybean oils).

Analysis of 'various ethnic populations' health over the past few decades has shown that since traditional saturated cooking fats have been replaced by polyunsaturated fats there have been significant increases in heart disease and diabetes in these populations.[32 33]

Stop using cooking oils to cook with. If you absolutely must cook with a fat then use **extra virgin coconut oil** to do so. Non-virgin coconut oil does not have the health benefits of cold-pressed virgin coconut oil so do not waste money on it.

Use moderate amounts of **monounsaturated** fats (extra virgin olive oil) as salad dressing only. Do not cook with it.

Omega-6 fats should come from natural dietary sources such as seeds and nuts. No cooking oils allowed!

Omega-3 fats should come from marine sources such as wild caught fatty fish or fish / krill oil supplements.

Saturated fat from of virgin coconut oil may be beneficial in small amounts.

8: PROTEIN

You need to dramatically cut down on your protein intake particularly if you eat animal protein. Most of us get far too much animal protein far too often. In fact some of us eat more protein daily than some professional athletes. This puts the kidneys under pressure. Our systems are not able to cope with all this extra stress on an already overloaded underactive metabolism

If you are eating fatty animal proteins then you will have weight gain issues to deal with also. We are at risk of cancer and heart disease when we consume too much animal protein. I will cover protein intake in greater detail in the next section.

9: NICOTINE [34]

Apart from the obvious reasons like cancer and emphysema women who smoke during pregnancy are more likely to produce children who will have diabetes hypertension and obesity. This may be from chromosomal damage or it may be learned behaviour, or a combination of both.

Nicotine also interferes with proper liver function causes vascular stenosis (narrowing of the arteries) chronic obstructive pulmonary disease (COPD) and emphysema and pneumonia.

In case you didn't get it, smoking damages blood vessels and arteries!

Nicotine is a known vasoconstrictor. Constricted arteries mean that there is less oxygenated blood flowing to limbs and organs. The heart has to work harder and there is a greater risk of heart disease. Your skin ages faster because there is less oxygenated blood reaching it and there is less elastin to keep it wrinkle-free. Nicotine is believed to stimulate the release of stored fat and cholesterol into the blood.

Smokers also require more vitamin C vitamin E vitamin D and calcium. Smoking lowers HDL (good) cholesterol and forms oxidized LDL cholesterol which contributes to the development of atherosclerosis. These are issues that someone with a metabolic disorder does not need to make any worse.

Stop using any nicotine as soon as possible. That means patches gum tobacco and electronic cigarettes.

10: ALCOHOL

1 can of beer has the same calorie content as 1 can of soda. That is 92 calories per can that will end up as fat just because you were thirsty. Most of do not stop at just one beer. 3 beers will amount to 276 calories which are consumed with the greatest of ease.

That being said there is evidence to support the enjoyment of one glass of red wine or one serving of any alcohol for that matter per day to reduce cholesterol levels. If you have the willpower to only have one drink per day then enjoy it for the medicinal value it provides.

Don't drink calories.

11: SWEETENERS

Some artificial sweeteners are excitotoxic, meaning that they destroy nerve cells. They all have long lists of side effects and some are even carcinogenic. There is new research that suggests that some artificial sweeteners stimulate appetite, carbohydrate cravings and fat storage.

Natural sweeteners may come from natural sources but they come with their own set of risks. Some of these natural sweeteners are marketed as low G,I which they are, but this is because they contain high levels of fructose which is the same as poison to a diabetic.

Some of the sugar-alcohol sugar substitutes will cause gastric distress if you take in too much over the course of the day.

Trying to fool yourself by using sweeteners of any kind can lead you consume more food under the belief that it is safe to do so. It is not. Go cold turkey and get off the sugars. All of them!

A WORD ON DIABETES

Type 2 Diabetes is a complicated metabolic disorder. At first glance there does not appear to be any medical cure for this disease and to be fair there isn't one. It is a "lifestyle" cure. Diet and exercise are the new medications.

We tend to look for the easy way out but in this case there is none. To succeed in this endeavour we are going to have to rethink everything we do. What we eat when we eat how we eat our physical activity levels everything.

If you fear change or it seems too challenging then take it one step at a time until you find it easy. It will happen.

MY MISTAKE: I thought that by choosing low fat and sugar free options my choices would have a dramatic effect on my diabetes. Imagine how disappointed I was when I was told my blood tests were still getting worse. I had been told to eat low fat foods and to eat less food and had been following the guidelines given to me by the diabetes association. I was doing something wrong and I had to find out what it was.

After doing exhaustive research I came to realise that it had more to do with what my food was than what was not in it. Refined anything is bad! Natural organic unprocessed wholefood is the only thing that is going to cure you! A low fat tortilla is still a refined flour tortilla. Skim milk is still a dairy product. I was not eating the right types of foods enough raw foods or enough unprocessed foods. I needed high fibre low GI / GL and a lot more vegetables in my diet.

I was not eating the types of foods that had the right ingredients in them to repair my system. I had been eating the same refined high carbohydrate foods as I was before only now they were low fat. I was drinking sugar free soda and using artificial sweetener in my coffee. I was drinking more fruit juice, up to a litre per day, in the belief that it was a healthy choice loaded with vitamins.

These were steps in the right direction but I was still not there yet. I needed to learn what real food and nutrition was. A sad fact that I learned was that the institutions that were supposed to help me manage my diabetes were clueless as to what the correct diet was that a diabetic needed to follow.

Perhaps it was beaurocratic nonsense, perhaps it was an inability to accept the proof of people who have reversed diabetes, I do not know. Many institutions whose job it is to assist diabetics with managing their diabetes are sadly keeping these very diabetics in a diabetic state with the advice and guidelines they are recommending.

Diabetes is a very lucrative business. With a huge percentage of the global population either diagnosed with diabetes or soon to be diagnosed with it there is a fortune to be made on medicating the various illnesses that develop as the disease progresses.

Diabetics can live for many years before the disease takes them and those years add up to a large amount of money spent on many different medications for many different symptoms and illnesses.

You don't make money by telling people to eat more vegetables! Money spent researching a cure for diabetes is not going to be recouped by advising a vegetable based diet and some exercise.

If you want to get off medications, and that should be your goal, then you will need to make serious lifestyle changes. These changes need to encompass diet, exercise and attitude to be successful.

START DOING THIS NOW!

1. Drink between 6-9 glasses of filtered **water** per day.

2. Eat more **raw food**. Aim for 80% total daily intake.

3. Adjust your **protein** intake.

4. Eat plenty of non-starchy low GI **vegetables** and **leafy greens.**

5. Eat more **nuts seeds berries** and some **pulses** and **legumes.**

6. Start **exercising** with particular emphasis on weight resistance exercises.

7. Drink **raw vegetable juices**.

8. Eat foods rich in healthy fats like **omega-3.**

9. Purchase **fresh organic** produce whenever possible.

10. Add more fibre to your diet.

11. Eat 3 regular meals per day. Do not skip meals.

1: WATER

The human body is 64 % water. A 70 kg man has 40 litres of water in total body matter averaging 60 % total weight. In infants this can be up to 75%. Old age and obesity decrease this amount. Obesity can lower it to an unhealthy 45%. Water makes up 75% of the brain (a percentage of fat is made up of water too) 83% of the blood 22% of the bones and 75% of the muscles.

Filtered water should be the only thing you consider drinking. Tap water contains fluoride which is a cause for hypothyroidism. It also poisons enzymes in the body raising the risks of cancer, bone diseases and seizures amongst others. High levels of calcium and magnesium in tap water has been shown to be goitrogenic (goitre causing).

Water is vital to the proper functioning of all systems in the body including cellular hydration nutrient transportation toxin removal regulating body temperature and healthy bowel movements. It is vitally important to a healthy metabolism and will help increase your resting metabolic rate. No water means no working metabolism.

Water is a basic natural element that the body cannot survive without. It is needed at the cellular level to sustain life. You die from thirst before you die from hunger.

You should be aiming for 6–9 glasses of filtered water per day. Tap water and bottled water have dissolved toxins in them from being treated and contained in plastic bottles or being carried for kilometres in pipes underground.

You are trying to detox and repair damaged cells so you do not need to add any more toxins to your system. Do not substitute with diet soda and absolutely do not substitute with fruit juice. These will need to be processed by the liver kidneys and digestive system before the water in them is extracted so you will have added more work for your already overworked liver and kidneys. The fructose in fruit juice also poses health risks.

Always keep water next to your bedside so that you can some if you get thirsty during the night. It should also be the first thing you drink in the morning. You've quit the caffeine remember? There are several herbal teas to consider as replacements for some of the water portions.

Consider rooibos tea or chai rooibos tea. They can be drunk unsweetened hot or cold, with or without lemon. Rooibos tea is caffeine free rich in anti-oxidants flavones and flavonols. Another tea with similar properties is honeybush tea. There are many available you will need to decide your preference. Try to drink herbal teas without sweeteners or milk added to them wherever possible. Sweetness and saltiness are both learned behaviour and can be un-learned.

Use glass or stainless steel containers to store your filtered water in. If you are exercising heavily and are sweating your daily water requirements may be more. If you cannot forgo juice then consider unsweetened juice that has been diluted by 1/3 to ½ with filtered water.

Natural coconut water is now available as a juice and is an excellent electrolyte. It was used during WWII as a blood substitute because it was sterile and had a perfect electrolyte ratio. It is high in potassium anti-oxidants and cytokinins which may have some health benefits and is also low in carbohydrates.

If you must have fruit juices then consider coconut water and fresh squeezed grapefruit juice as options. They have beneficial health properties. Be sure to enjoy them as treats only occasionally and not as everyday necessities.

2: RAW FOOD

Raw foods contain high concentrations of nutrients and fibre. Cooking destroys up to 50% of all the nutrition in food and this is even more so in processed foods. Cooking also significantly raises the GI of food. This means your food now has less protein and nutrients and it will also significantly raise your blood glucose levels

Cooking will destroy valuable enzymes in foods too. Enzymes help to digest food to carry toxins away to support the endocrine system to transport nutrients and hormones and many other functions.

There is a correlation to be made between the prevalence of disease in our society and the amount of enzyme poor food that we eat.

Try to aim for at least 80 % of your daily food intake to be raw.

3: PROTEIN

Our bodies are 22% protein and we need quality protein to regenerate and replace our damaged cells. Proteins are made up of 21 different amino acids of which the body is only capable of producing 13 of   these are non- essential amino acids the remaining 9 called essential amino acids need to come from our diet. We still need to consume foods that contain the non-essential amino acids.

Proteins that lack one or more essential amino acids are called incomplete proteins. Beans grains nuts fruits and vegetables are examples of incomplete proteins. This does not really matter since a well-balanced diet will contain foods that have the needed amino acids to complete the protein.

As long as you get all the amino acids in one day you will be able to create protein. It does not have to come from one single source i.e. animal protein since we are able to get protein from vegetable sources too. Leafy green vegetables have an excellent amino acid profile i.e. protein.

Chlorella and spirulina are both vegetables high in protein. Yellow peas, brown rice, sacha inchi and hemp seeds are all now being used to extract vegetarian protein for use as protein supplements. A substances' protein content is all about the amino acid profile of that substance

Be aware that some vegetable protein supplements may cause problems when used excessively. I developed high uric acid levels when using pea protein concentrate daily for a number of months. Peas contain a high purine content which leads to high uric acid levels.

It is advised that you use a selection of vegetarian protein powders to get a broad amino acid profile as single sources of protein will be limited in terms of their total amino acid profile.

There is a lot of debate over the bio-availability of certain vegetable proteins. This is of little concern. As long as all the necessary amino acids are available they will be utilised to create protein within the body.

If anyone is in doubt about vegetarian muscle then do some research on Bill Pearl, who was born in 1930, went ovo-vegetarian in 1969 because too much red meat was endangering his health. The man is a legend in the bodybuilding fraternity. There are many other vegetarian bodybuilders who disprove the myth. Do some research on Robert Cheeke, Danny Dalton, Joel Kirkilis and Albert Beckles if you need visual confirmation that vegetarians can grow big muscle.

You need a daily supply of all the amino acids to make protein because the body doesn't store amino acids like it does fats or carbohydrates. If we don't consume enough protein in our diet the body will use the only available source our muscle tissue to get what it needs. It is for this reason that many people have argued against vegan diets citing poor health. Their diets were not varied enough and they were not getting adequate nutrition from a wide enough variety of foods.

Less muscle tissue further contributes to a slowed metabolism and reduced fat-burning.

Unless you are an athlete training for a competition or an event chances are good that you are getting far too much animal protein in your diet. Athletes need about 2.4g of protein per kg of bodyweight per day and non-athletes only need 0.9g of protein per kilogram of bodyweight per day. For women this would be around 70g per day in total and for men it should be around 100g per day in total. Not much at all if you are not exercising.

Your protein requirements will depend on your bodyweight and whether or not you are exercising heavily. If you are exercising moderate too heavily you will need more protein to repair muscle tissue. If you are not exercising or are doing light exercise such as yoga or walking you may not need to supplement with protein at all.

These are rough estimates only and your own discretion is advised when planning your daily meals. Vegetarians and vegans will have different requirements for protein.

The kidneys are responsible for excreting urea formed from ammonia by a diet high in animal protein. This is bad news for the kidneys. You should consider cutting down your meat chicken and fish portion sizes by quite a bit if you do eat meat.

The liver is only able to metabolise 200g-300 g of animal protein per day. Most of us consume this amount sometimes more than once a day every day. This sort of massive animal protein consumption causes the production of toxins which need to be removed. If they are not removed they build up and cause health issues.

A diet high in animal protein can in fact cause protein deficiency due to pancreatic overload but this would be an extreme situation. Diets high in animal protein also increase your risk of colon cancer prostate cancer and osteoporosis.

The pancreas produces proteolytic enzymes to break down proteins into amino acids. An overloaded pancreas does not produce enough proteolytic enzymes which can lead to undigested protein molecules being absorbed into the bloodstream and that in turn causes inflammation. A similar thing happens with milk protein in infants that can cause type 1 diabetes.

Excessive consumption of fatty animal protein increases the production of homocysteine (used to transform protein). Excess homocysteine in the blood causes damage to the tissues of the Arteries (causing heart attacks and strokes), the Brain (causing Alzheimer's disease), the bones (causing osteoporosis) and the DNA (causing cancer).

Excess unused protein has a tendency to bind with minerals creating nutrient deficiencies. An increase in a waste product called urea leads to dehydration and high acidity levels in the body which are bad.

The liver and kidneys are put under strain trying to remove excess waste making kidney disease a real possibility. Another thing to remember is that the human body operates better in alkaline conditions and animal protein consumption turns that into an acidic environment.

These are all possibilities just from excess animal protein consumption. The problem gets worse when saturated animal fat is added into the equation.

If you do not want to go vegetarian you must at least consider cutting your animal protein intake drastically. I am not a vegetarian and would find it difficult to become one but I have learned to be more reserved about my animal protein intake. Do not misunderstand me we definitely need protein in our diets but animal protein is not the only source of protein. If you do not intend to become a full vegetarian and I personally chose not to you will need to make your meat portions much smaller and less frequent. Consider only having 2 to 3 meat-containing meals per week maximum out of 21 potential meals per week.

Animal proteins contain Vitamin B12 and heme iron not found in vegetables and for this reason I did not consider becoming a complete vegetarian. This was my personal choice you decide for yourself. If you do decide to eat meat remember to eat less, less often. Since you will be eating less meat you can spend more on better quality organic free range produce which will be healthier for you.

If you choose to be vegetarian you are on the right track to health. Keep an eye on your vitamin B12 levels and make sure you supplement well for a broad spectrum of omega 3 fatty acids and vitamin D.

CAUTION:

if you are a vegetarian who is exercising moderately to heavily you need to ensure a sufficient protein intake or you will develop serious health issues. Protein is required for energy and repair and exercise place a demand for protein on the body.

There are vegetarian non-dairy protein powders available but make sure that you consult a nutritionist to calculate your protein requirements based on body weight exercise levels and type of diet.

Not enough is as bad as too much of the wrong sort of protein, as I found out when my uric acid levels went too high for comfort, after adding pea protein to my morning breakfast smoothies.

Be wary of some protein sources that may appear to be healthy. Veal may be lower in fat than beef but it has a higher cholesterol level than beef as do many other animal proteins like shrimp.

While salmon may contain healthy omega 3 fatty acids, it also has a high purine content which could lead to gout so be aware of this too. You can eat too much of a good thing.

Limit animal proteins to only a few times per week if you must eat animal protein.

RABBIT STARVATION

Eating lean animal protein can also have its consequences. A strange phenomenon known as rabbit starvation (aka protein poisoning or mal de caribou) occurs when humans survive on nothing but lean animal protein for an extended period of time without any other food sources being available.

It is a form of starvation in which the body does not get enough nutrients despite large amounts of lean protein being consumed.
This does not occur if fatty animal protein is consumed instead.

I include this here as an example that even apparently healthy foods can have negative impacts if consumed to excess. We are a concentrate selective omnivore species.

We thrive on small amounts of nutrient dense foods from a wide variety of sources. Relying too much on one food source causes imbalance and disease.

Make certain that your diet is varied and contains plenty of fibre and nutrient dense vegetables and some fats, both saturated and mono-unsaturated.

4: VEGETABLES

When you go to the supermarket pay attention to what is at the entrance and around the outskirts as opposed to what is in the isles of the supermarket. You are being marketed psychologically targeted while shopping.

The vegetables are located near the entrance so that once you have chosen your healthy foods you no longer feel guilty about buying unhealthy treats snacks and convenience foods in the isles. This is a deliberate industrial psychology tool employed against you the consumer! Be aware of this and shop the outskirts of the store not the isles. Use a shopping list that you do not deviate from.

Leafy green vegetables brightly coloured vegetables cruciferous vegetables and salads should be made the cornerstone of your diet if you truly want to beat this disease! You should avoid starchy vegetables like potato and be cautious with vegetables like kumara sweet potato and pumpkin.

We should all be aiming for at least 1Lb / 500g each per day of raw leafy greens. That is a hefty amount which I am not able to do but still attempt. You can eat this as a salad or drink it as a green smoothie the choice is yours so long as it is raw. Victoria Boutenko is an author and raw food advocate who wrote "Green for Life". In the book she lists the nutritional components in leafy green vegetables. They are a near perfect match for the nutritional requirements for humans.

We need to concentrate on leafy greens and brightly coloured non-starchy vegetables. These are vegetables that have high nutritional value loaded with vitamins minerals fibre and phytonutrients. Consistent daily consumption of raw leafy green vegetables will help to lower your HbA1c levels over time.

Some vegetables to consider adding to your diet are; green beans (string beans), broccoli, brussel sprouts, cabbage, spinach, kale, bok choy, pak choy, collard greens (bore-kale), Romaine lettuce(cos), onions, garlic, ginger, chillies, chives, spring onions, celery, cucumber, capsicum, tomatoes, asparagus, bitter melon, okra, avocado and all salad leaves. All cruciferous vegetables are acceptable. Cruciferous vegetables like cabbage, brussel sprouts, kale, broccoli etc. help to improve liver function. Remember to rotate your vegetables and do not eat too much of any one thing too often.

Raw vegetables green smoothies and raw vegetable juices should account for at least 60-80% of your food intake. This may sound crazy but it is a proven method for reversing diabetes. The nutrient and fibre content of raw vegetables is unmatched by cooked food. Cooking destroys up to 50% of all the nutrients in vegetables and raises the GI.

You need to eat protein with carbohydrates to slow down the conversion to glucose so if you do eat something starchy it needs to be combined with protein and fibre. Lemon juice, lime juice and vinegar have also been shown to slow down the absorption of carbohydrates so add a splash of balsamic or lemon juice to your vegetables or salad. Fibre does the same job if you are not a big fan of acidic foods.

MY MISTAKE: During my dietary intervention I was consuming more fruit and fruit juice under the mistaken belief that this was healthier. It was no surprise then that my test results were worse than ever. I was taking in more of the poison that caused my diabetes.

I believe that 1-2 pieces of fruit per week max is acceptable and even healthy, but no more than that and definitely no fruit juice. (I make the exception for home-made green apple juice occasionally due to its high malic acid content and grapefruit juice which has benefits relating to glucose absorption) Notice that I used the word **occasionally**. Remember that fructose is poison!

When I switched to raw vegetable juices I noticed a distinct improvement in my health. Some foods appear to have more benefit for diabetics than others due to their specific phytonutrient content.

The long-term consumption of high GL foods is associated with type 2 diabetes and coronary heart disease. There is a greater risk of cancer with a high GI diet as cancer cells thrive on glucose.

Some foods may have a high GI but a low GL. Watermelon for example has a high GI (it is a fast releasing carbohydrate) of 72 but has a low GL (there is very little carbohydrate in 120g) of only 4 points. This means that while you may have been told to stay away from watermelon because of its high GI (which is true) you would have to eat large amounts of it to have a drastic effect on your blood glucose levels. A 120g serving of watermelon has only 6g of carbohydrate.

Starchy vegetables will be quickly converted into glucose. Leafy green vegetables and most other vegetables may be eaten raw. This will give you more fibre and more nutrients without raising your blood glucose levels too much.

5: FRUITS NUTS SEEDS AND BERRIES

Fruits should generally be avoided as the fructose content should be avoided at all cost. Sour green apples are a rich source of malic acid which is a good anti-inflammatory and helps lower blood pressure so I chose to eat small amounts of them occasionally as a snack with nuts. I did occasionally add them to green juices to make them more palatable.

Some fruits are high in enzymes that are beneficial. Pineapple has bromelain a proteolytic enzyme (protein digesting) kiwifruit has actinidin (protease) and pawpaw (papaya) has papain (protease). Berries are a rich source of antioxidants to help fight the oxidative tissue damage that is present in diabetes and are good for breakfast smoothies.

The occasional piece of fruit in a smoothie or as a treat is acceptable as long as fruit is not a daily occurrence. Fruit is seasonal and our ancestors did not eat fruit daily. Our bodies are not able to cope with vast amounts of fruit on a daily basis all year long and most definitely not concentrated fruit juice. Fruit should always be consumed whole and not as a fibreless concentrated juice. The fibre plays an important part in how the fructose is metabolised.

Berries like blueberries are a good source of anti-oxidants and other phytochemicals. Use them in smoothies or salads or as a snack but be cautious with dried berries as they are often treated with sugar and vegetable oil.

Nuts and seeds provide protein and fibre and are a valuable source of all the omega fatty acids that we need for good heart and brain functioning and to prevent inflammation.

7: RAW VEGETABLE JUICES

Raw vegetable juices are a good source of concentrated vitamins, minerals, enzymes, fibre and phytonutrients. Do some research to find out which vegetables are best suited to your particular needs Be careful not to include fruits as this will add unwanted fructose to your juice.

http://www.rebootwithjoe.com/about/fat-sick-and-nearly-dead/

ENZYMES

Enzymes are protein molecules and ninety-eight of the 5000 known so far have been found in in the arteries. The there is a theory that over 100 000 enzymes are needed for the maintenance of a healthy body. They are crucial to healing digestion and metabolism.

Many fruits and vegetables and juices available on the supermarket shelves have had their enzymes destroyed by pasteurising or irradiation. These products will have a much longer shelf life but will now cause the pancreas to work harder to produce enzymes needed to replace the destroyed enzymes.

Cooking food also causes the destruction of enzymes and once again the pancreas will need to work harder to produce enzymes. Studies have shown that diets high in cooked foods cause the pancreas to enlarge over time. As the pancreas deteriorates over time it produces less enzymes and that leads to disease and illness.

Eating more raw foods and drinking lots of raw vegetable juice daily will ensure that you get an adequate supply of vitamins minerals and enzymes. There will be less stress put on your pancreas and your body should heal faster.

8: OMEGA-3-6-9 FATTY ACIDS

The human brain is 60% fat. We need fat! It is crucial to our survival but it has to be the right sort of fat I the right amount. Walnut oil macadamia nut oil flax (linseed) oil extra virgin olive oil ground flax seed and chia seeds are excellent sources of omega-3 and omega-6 polyunsaturated fats. These are not to be used in cooking however.

Nuts and seeds provide both protein and healthy fats rich in omega-3 and omega-6. Be cautious of having too much omega-6 fat as it can lead to inflammation if consumed in excess.

Add raw walnuts, almonds, sunflower seeds, avocadoes and pumpkin seeds to your meals.

Food cooked in vegetable oil tends to be high in omega 6 fatty acid that along with the production of AGEs is why fried foods are so bad for us. Our modern diet also contains way too much omega-6 oils which are found in everything processed.

A good ratio of omega 6 to omega 3 fatty acids is 2:1 and can be found occurring naturally in flaxseed oil. Our average today is 20:1 and has been used as an explanation for the meteoric rise in obesity diabetes and other serious health issues.

We need omega-6 fatty acids to be healthy but we are getting ten times the amount we actually need. Stop using cooking oils for cooking. Choose the best quality cold pressed oils you can afford and use them sparingly as dressings for salads.

8: OMEGA-3 FATTY ACIDS

Omega 3 fatty acids are polyunsaturated fats found in marine and plant oils and organic free range chicken eggs. They are essential fatty acids which cannot be made in the body and need to come from our diet.

They have been used in the treatment of cancer inflammation developmental disorders psychiatric disorders and cardiovascular disease. Omega-3 PUFA reduces the production of TNF and IL-6 from fat cells. These are the main causes for inflammation so make sure that you have a daily dose of omega-3s. They are also believed to help reduce insulin resistance. There are several omega 3 fatty acids but the 3most important ones for us are:

8.1: DHA (DOCOSAHEXAENOIC ACID) a

marine sourced omega-3 fatty acid that has been shown to reduce blood levels of triglycerides and thereby reduce the risk of heart disease. DHA levels have been shown to be low in patients with ADD and Alzheimer's disease and supplementation with DHA has shown some improvement in patients. 40% of the polyunsaturated fatty acid in the brain is made from DHA. DHA is a primary structural component of the cerebral cortex sperm testicles and retina.

DHA in supplement form can be found in fish oil krill oil or in algae based capsules or synthesized from alpha-linolenic acid. In food it can be found in cold water fatty fish like salmon, herring, sardines and albacore or Bluefin tuna or from seaweed.

DHA reduces inflammation blood pressure triglycerides and arterial plaque formation.

8.2: EPA (EICOSAPENTAENOIC ACID):
the other most common omega 3 fatty acid found in **marine food sources**. Supplementing with EPA has shown dramatic improvements in mental health in test patients. It promotes healthy cholesterol and triglyceride levels. Both DHA and EPA are found in the same sources and generally have the same health benefits attributed to them. They are 2 of several omega 3 fatty acids.

8.3: ALA (ALPHA-LINOLENIC ACID): is
another omega 3 fatty acid but is derived from **plant sources** such as walnuts hemp seed/oil chia seeds and linseed (flaxseed). ALA is the "mother "fatty acid to EPA and DHA and can be converted to either if need be albeit in small amounts.

ALA is believed to control blood clotting build cell membranes in the brain and reduces inflammation. It is used to treat joint pain and stiffness and improve mobility in patients with arthritis. It may also help to treat diseases such as lupus and assist asthma sufferers by improving lung function and decreasing inflammation.

Because only small trace amounts of EPA and DHA are actually created from ALA it is necessary to supplement with **marine fish oil supplements** to get the benefit of all 3of these omega 3 fatty acids. DHA and EPA are best derived from marine sources while ALA is best from plant sources like flax walnuts sesame seeds and sunflower seeds.

SIDE NOTE: alpha-lipoic acid is sometimes abbreviated as ALA. Alpha-lipoic acid is an antioxidant that converts glucose into energy and should not be mistaken for Alpha-Linolenic Acid.

CAUTION: animal studies in Canada have shown that diets containing high levels of linolenic acid may cause cardiac tissue necrosis (the death of heart muscle tissue).
Get your ALA from nuts and seeds. Do not use vegetable oils (except extra virgin olive oil). If you do choose to use them, then use them sparingly.

We have all been convinced that certain oils are safe to use because they are not saturated and supposedly heart-safe, but they appear to have the same effect in the long term.

OMEGA-6 FATTY ACIDS

Omega-6 fatty acids are unsaturated fatty acids of which there are several such as Gamma-linolenic acid (GLA) Linolenic acid (LA) and Arachidonic acid (AA). These are found in many of the vegetable oils we consume such as sunflower, cottonseed, canola and corn. Omega-6 fatty acids have similar health benefits to omega-3 fatty acids however high levels of omega-6 will actually cause disease.

Eicosanoids produced by excessively high levels of omeg-6 have been linked to arthritis inflammation and cancer. We need omega-6 fatty acids in our diet but we often consume up to 30x the amount we actually need.

OMEGA-9 FATTY ACIDS

Omega-9 fatty acids are unsaturated fatty acids found in vegetable and animal fats. They are not essential fatty acids like omega-3 and omega-9 fatty acids because our bodies are able to create them form unsaturated fat

Omega-9 fatty acids are the most abundant of all the omega fatty acids. When our diets lack sufficient omega-3 and omega-6 our bodies try to compensate by creating extra omega-9 fatty acids.

They help to lower the risk of cardiovascular disease and stroke.

9: ORGANIC FOOD

Organic foods whether animal vegetable or mineral should have as little added to them as possible either to make them grow bigger more in quantity or to prevent diseases and pests from bothering them. They should be as close to pure as possible and that means they will have blemishes so deal with it!

Our food is intended to supply us with all the nutrition our bodies require and not just to look good while it sits on the shelf.

Try shopping at local farmer's markets instead of buying imported foods that have been treated with gases to keep them from going bad during transport.

SIDE NOTE: Foods imported from other countries will often be subjected to chemical treatments to prevent any foreign pests or diseases from contaminating the domestic food supply. This renders the organic label void.

Buying local produce ensures consumption of a more nutritionally dense seasonal foodstuff. It may not look as pretty as the stuff in the supermarket but it is a lot more nutritious. Imported frozen goods are acceptable as freezing locks in the nutrition just make sure that it is **organic** frozen produce.

Organic locally grown foods will be fresher and more nutritious than imported foods that have been in storage for extended periods of time and will have a stronger natural resistance to diseases and infections since they are not reliant on pesticides and introduced chemicals. This translates into more naturally occurring phytochemicals which are of benefit to us.

The produce available at a local farmer's market or organic store will also teach you about seasonal foods i.e. what grows when and where it comes from in your particular region. Fruits and vegetables are seasonal or at least they used to be. We now eat fruits and vegetables out of season in quantities that our bodies have not yet evolved to cope with.

The human body has evolved over centuries to eat foods as they appear in season. We have changed that pattern. Is it any wonder that we now have so many metabolic diseases to plague us?

10: FIBRE

Fibre plays an important role in insulin sensitivity and weight management. It reduces the rate at which sugar is absorbed into the blood from the gut which means less sugar turns into fructose which means less fructose turns into fat. Fibre helps to make you feel "fuller" sooner by speeding up digestion and stimulating Peptide YY (PYY) which send a signal to the brain that you are now full. Fibre helps to supress insulin secretion by transporting fats to the colon where bacteroides turn the fats into short chain fatty acids which supress insulin secretion as opposed to long chain fatty acids which stimulate the secretion of insulin.

There are two types of fibre found in our foods:

Soluble Fibre or **prebiotic fibre** is any fibre which absorbs water to become a gelatinous viscous substance that is then fermented in the colon to produce bioactive by-products beneficial to the body. Sources of soluble fibre are beans peas lentils chia seeds oats rye barley broccoli carrots nuts and root vegetables.

Insoluble Fibre is not digested or fermented at all. It acts as a bulking medium and as a sort of internal broom to sweep out garbage. Sources of insoluble fibre are nuts, flaxseeds, wholegrains, celery, avocado, green beans and the skins of tomatoes.

Soluble fibre binds to bile acids in the small intestine preventing them from entering the body and thereby lowering cholesterol. Soluble fibre reduces both the absorption of and response to sugar in the system.

Fibre helps to regulate our blood glucose levels and to remove toxins from our bodies. Our ancestors consumed as much as 100g of fibre per day. The daily average in our world is between 10-12 g per day. We should be aiming for a minimum of 50g per day.

There are fibre supplements available if you feel you are not getting enough in your diet. Adding a tablespoon of ground flaxseed/linseed to your meals is a good way to start. This will also add beneficial omega3s to your diet.

Everybody has heard the sermon about needing more fibre in their diet. Not many of us know why it is so important so here's why.

- Fibre slows down the rate at which carbohydrates are absorbed and so minimizes the insulin response.
- Fibre helps to remove toxins from the body.
- Fibre inhibits the absorption of some free fatty acids (FFA) which would otherwise be metabolised into short chain fatty acids (SCFA) which suppress insulin.
- Fibre stimulates the release of Peptide YY (the satiety hormone) which lets your brain know that you are full.

When we eat fibreless refined carbohydrates like white rice or white sugar they get absorbed too fast. The liver becomes overloaded and the mitochondria stop working correctly. You now have insulin resistance. Fibre prevents this from happening.

BETA-GLUCANS: These are polysaccharides or soluble fibres found in baker's yeast, oats, oat bran, barley bran, Reishi mushroom, Shiitake mushroom and Maitake mushroom and some types of seaweed. Beta glucans are

150

called biological response modifiers because of their ability to activate the immune system. A receptor on the surface of immune cells called Complement Receptor 3 (CR3 or CD11b/CD18) is responsible for binding to beta glucans allowing the immune cells to recognize them as non-self. There is also scientific evidence to link regular consumption of beta-glucans with normal healthy cholesterol levels[35].

INULIN: This type of soluble fibre that belongs to a class called fructans. It is not digested by the gastrointestinal tract but is fermented by intestinal flora in the large intestine. This is makes it both a pre-biotic and a fibre supplement.

It is commonly found in roots and rhizomes like chicory onions jicama Jerusalem artichoke garlic and yams. It is thought to help lower cholesterol and glucose levels. It also helps to increase bone density by improving calcium absorption. The best part is that it is sweet and is used as a sugar substitute.

If you do decide to try inulin be warned that too much will cause intestinal distress.

11: 3 MEALS A DAY

Eating 3 regular meals per day will help to keep good control over blood glucose levels. It will also keep your leptin and ghrelin levels under control. If these 2 hormones are working efficiently then you are well on your way to getting better. Eating 3 nutrient dense, phytochemical rich meals a day will ensure a constant supply of the good stuff to ensure that internal repair work gets done.

Do not snack between meals as this interferes with the way that leptin and ghrelin work. Try to make sure that your 3 meals per day are sufficient enough to keep you from getting hungry between meals. A healthy vegan diet will exclude you from having to worry about calorie-counting.

Hunger pains lead to snacking and this is where it all starts to go wrong. Drink water or a calorie free beverage like decaffeinated green tea if you are feeling hungry.

Do not skip meals if at all possible as this can interfere with thyroid hormone production and your body goes into "fasting" mode.

LEPTIN

Leptin is known as the appetite hormone. Its purpose is to suppress your appetite when you have reached satiety. It is produced by fat cells and acts on receptors in the hypothalamus where it inhibits appetite. It counters the effects of the feeding stimulants Neuropeptide Y and Anandamide.

The body's fat cells produce the hormone Leptin to tell the brain that we are full. It also tells the body that we have enough energy to exercise. A lack of leptin or leptin receptors will cause uncontrolled eating. When the brain cannot register leptin it assumes that we are starving and keeps us hungry. We lose the urge to exercise and we get fat.

Sugar is an appetite stimulant. It causes you to eat more. It also causes a rise in insulin levels. High insulin levels make you feel hungry so you again you eat more. Add this to the fact that the brain cannot see leptin and you have high insulin levels and you have a big problem on your hands. Remember that insulin is a fat storage hormone.

Refined carbohydrates sugar and fructose cause large amounts of leptin to be released. Over time our brain becomes resistant to these high levels of leptin and leptin resistance arises.

Leptin resistance and insulin resistance are closely related. In a strange twist of fate the more overweight you are the more leptin you have in circulation and the more resistant you will be to its appetite suppressing effects.

Leptin is made from white adipose tissue. WAT is the bad fat around our bellies that we are trying to lose and the more WAT we make the more leptin we make.

This might sound good but not if we are resistant to its effect. Research has also shown that high leptin levels correlate with cravings for alcohol. Stress, lack of exercise, high fructose intake and high GI diets also contribute to leptin resistance.

Diets high in starchy carbohydrates and any high GI carbohydrates should be avoided at all costs to prevent leptin resistance.

The rules for good leptin management:

1. Eat a high protein breakfast.
2. Eat 3 meals per day absolutely no snacking between meals.
3. Do not eat large meals.
4. Eat slowly chewing thoroughly.
5. Reduce refined carbohydrate intake dramatically.
6. Avoid processed foods completely.

Following a high fibre low GI / GL diet and doing regular daily exercise will assist in weight loss and bring leptin resistance under control. Sleep improves leptin sensitivity so make sure that you get enough sleep and stop eating sugar.

GHRELIN

Ghrelin is an appetite stimulating peptide hormone the hunger hormone. It is the counterpart to leptin and is produced in the stomach and stimulates the hypothalamus into generating appetite. In a normal functioning metabolism Ghrelin levels increase before a meal and decrease after a meal.

It plays a significant role in learning and adapting to changing environments and defends against stress-induced depression and anxiety. Ghrelin stimulates the pituitary gland to produce growth hormone. These are good points but ghrelin also stimulates lipid (fat) retention. It specifically targets the retention of belly fat the worst kind as belly fat is linked to liver fat.

Research has shown that not getting adequate sleep will reduce leptin levels (the appetite suppressant) and increase ghrelin levels (the appetite stimulant). This can potentially cause increased appetite and therefore obesity. Obese people have lower ghrelin levels than lean people.

Make sure you get enough sleep!

Ghrelin also stimulates the appetite for high calorie foods when you are hungry or have skipped a meal so do not skip meals, especially breakfast.

NOTES

STRESS

"Stress is the trash of modern life-we all generate it but if you don't dispose of it properly it will pile up and overtake your life."
— *Danzae Pace*

THE 2 TYPES OF STRESS

EUSTRESS: *Positive motivational stress.*

DISTRESS: *Negative destructive stress.*

"Every stress leaves an indelible scar and the organism pays for its survival after a stressful situation by becoming a little older."
-Hans Selye

Endocrinologist Hans Selye coined the term Eustress to describe the positive form of stress. When you win the lottery or a competition etc. this would be stressful but in a good way i.e. eustress. Distress is the negative side of the coin and the one we are all more familiar with like when you crash the car.

Stress is the physical manifestation of our psychological reaction to an event. The way in which we perceive an event will cause hormonal reactions which will then stimulate physical reactions. If the perception is negative then the hormones released in response to this will stress hormones and not the hormones associated with love or happiness. No really!

We find ourselves more stressed than ever before and more unable to deal with the things that stress us often unaware of what these stressors are. To make matters worse we over-use stimulants and watch adrenaline releasing movies sports or events on a daily basis. We are burning out our hormone producing organs faster than ever before. We are aging faster.

The problem with stress is that it is cumulative i.e. the more you stress the more you stay stressed. Sugar caffeine alcohol and food additives can all increase stress levels so make sure that you pay close attention to your diet.

HOW DO YOU KNOW YOU ARE STRESSED?
Do you experience "brain fog" get irritable easily lose your temper over simple things get panic attacks find it difficult to get out of bed find it difficult to get to sleep get regular headaches and sweat too much? Are you forgetful and un-focussed? Are you putting on weight around your belly? Do you have a continuous dialogue going on inside your head? Do you get facial tics or twitches? Do your eyes quiver or twitch?

You are stressed!

With your blood sugar going up and down you will be experiencing the "highs" and the "crashes". This inevitably leads to using stimulants and eating the wrong types of food as a means of compensating. Sugar affects the reward centre of the brain so you may find yourself craving sweet things when stressed.

ADRENAL FATIGUE

The adrenal glands are two triangular glands that sit on top of the kidneys. They are responsible for dealing with physical stress emotional stress infections and inflammation. Emotional stressors as well as physical stressors will affect your adrenal glands. Sugar is an example of a physical stressor that wears down the adrenal glands.

After many years of continuous exposure to stress and stimulants and sugar your adrenal glands will have worn out. They will have burnt out by being expected to pump out massive doses of cortisol and adrenaline on a daily basis.

The symptoms of adrenal stress include dizziness, headaches, fatigue, mood swings and trouble sleeping.

Adrenal fatigue affects cognition too. Neural excitability is a survival mechanism. Your brain is continuously switched on trying to find a solution to whatever is stressing you. You have random thoughts coming at you constantly; it affects your focus your attention and your memory.

It will affect your tolerance levels too. You will have very little patience for anything that your brain considers non-essential for survival or that it perceives as a threat to your survival. You will find yourself getting angry and annoyed at many things people and situations without any real justification.

It will affect your sleep patterns too especially the circadian rhythms that occur during deep sleep. Deep sleep is the time the body uses to burn fat so if you are not sleeping well you are not burning fat i.e. you are getting fat.

Adrenal stress causes the loss of electrolytes like sodium and potassium. This causes a craving for salty foods. This can lead to overeating and cravings for junk food and high blood pressure if not kept in check.it can also lead to bradycardia (very low heart rate).

Adrenal fatigue is linked to high cholesterol heart disease diabetes allergies muscle atrophy fluid retention and acid reflux and a few other health issues.

CHOLESTEROL

Studies have shown that individuals who are exposed to chronic stress will have high cholesterol.[36] There are several theories as to why this is. One belief is that stress causes the body to produce more energy in the form of glucose or fatty acids for the fight or flight response. These require the liver to produce more LDL.

Another theory suggests that stress interfere with the normal lipid clearance. Stress also causes inflammatory compound like **TNF (Tumor Necrosis Factor) interleukin-6 (IL-6)** and **C-reactive protein**. [37]

The body also requires cholesterol for the production of stress hormones. If more stress hormones are needed then more cholesterol will be produced. Both adrenaline and cortisol trigger the production of cholesterol. Excess cholesterol in the system is easily converted to LDL cholesterol if the right conditions are met.

CORTISOL

Cortisol is THE stress hormone. Normal levels of cortisol prevent cell damage by protecting cells against toxic chemicals electrolyte imbalance and cellular dehydration auto-immune reactions inflammatory reactions high insulin levels and glucose deficiencies. It acts like a buffer against stress.

These are the functions of normal levels of cortisol in the blood. Abnormal levels will actually cause problems. Cortisol is the body's primary anti-inflammatory hormone. If you are exposed to stress on a daily basis for a many years your body will downgrade the receptors for cortisol.

This means that you will have high levels of cortisol in your blood which is not being used to treat inflammation. This leads to fibromyalgia which is basically inflammatory pain throughout the entire body. There is also the possibility of sinus infections occurring when the anti-inflammatory responses are down.

High blood insulin levels lead to a reduction in the production of serotonin (the feel-good hormone) which leads to increased cortisol levels. The depletion of serotonin causes depression which causes raised stress hormone levels (like cortisol) as a defence mechanism.

Neural excitability is an inability to switch off the thought process so you have a continuous internal dialogue going on inside your head which inevitably turns to bad thoughts i.e. stress or worrying. This is another side effect of cortisol resistance.

Cortisol is also catabolic (breaks down muscle tissue) hormone so muscle wasting is a possibility. Other issues to keep an eye open for include vitamin A deficiency systolic hypertension salt cravings sleep apnea and belly fat.

Cortisol is responsible for telling the body to store fat around the belly. This is called visceral fat and is the body's way of protecting the internal organs located around that area. It is a survival mechanism initiated during a time of stress.

High levels of cortisol can lead to high estrogen levels. This causes a hormonal imbalance that can lead to low levels of T3. Low levels of T3 can lead to hypothyroidism which means lowered immunity and weight gain.

It also causes the production of blood glucose just what every diabetic needs. This continuous exposure to stress causes continuous rises in blood glucose levels which become converted into triglycerides or fatty acids. This will become visceral (belly) fat and if you don't have it already diabetes and heart disease.

When we are under stress our bodies seem to crave certain types of food because cortisol stimulates the appetite. We crave foods that will give us energy to run away or to fight neither of which we do. We eat stodgy "comfort food" when we feel down and we use energy" drinks to perk us up. Our bodies crave salty high starch high sugar and high fat foods in an attempt to keep us well supplied with energy and electrolytes during our distress. We use stimulants to keep us awake and alert and in doing so we lose precious healing sleep.

When you are under stress, stress hormones like epinephrine (adrenaline) and cortisol kick in and stimulate the release of blood glucose. This is your body responding to the threat of danger and trying to make sure you have enough immediate energy to fight or run away. These are good if you are an athlete who is training or competing. If you are not running away or fighting or going to gym or using up all that excess blood glucose then you have a big problem.

Over a period of time while under stress your pituitary gland adrenal gland pancreas and liver are all pumping out hormones to release and control your blood glucose which isn't being used properly. All this energy is being diverted away from the body's normal repair processes.

Repair happens after the battle is over but we are constantly in "battle" mode with no repair time scheduled. Long term exposure to stress hormones is proven to suppress the immune system.

CARDIAC MUSCLE CATABOLISM

Catabolism occurs when proteins fats and polysaccharides are broken down by the body order to feed itself. It is in a sense self-cannibalism. Cortisol glucagon adrenalin e and cytokines are known catabolics.

Hormonal imbalances and chronic stress can also trigger a catabolic state. Diabetes is also connected with a type of cardiomyopathy that is not very well understood but what is known is that exposure to stress hormones dramatically increases your risk of contracting this type of cardiomyopathy. Cardiomyopathy is defined as a physical change in the structure and/or functioning of the heart.

Insulin is needed to regulate protein anabolism in both skeletal and heart muscles and low insulin levels appear to cause catabolism of the cardiac muscle proteins. Basically the heart atrophies due to insufficient protein availability.

In other words diabetes increases your risk of losing heart muscle protein which increases your risk of heart failure from contractile dysfunction not necessarily only from a stroke or coronary artery disease. Being exposed to low levels of insulin due to insulin resistance or not enough insulin being produced alongside high levels of stress released hormones will most certainly lead you to heart failure.

There is no treatment at present for this type of cardiomyopathy but supplementing with CoQ10 has been of great benefit in many other types of heart disease. Research has shown that patients with heart disease tend to be deficient in this particular nutrient.

P53

No it's not a drug. Long term exposure to adrenaline causes levels of a protein called P53, a tumour suppressor, to fall. P53, also called the Guardian of the Genome, allows DNA repair proteins to repair DNA when there is damage. This includes the cells that produce pigment in hair. Less P53 means more grey hair.

Prolonged exposure to high levels of adrenaline will drop the levels of p53 which will cause many other forms of damage not just grey hair. P53 is known primarily as an anti-cancer gene but it also helps controls glucose metabolism. It binds to and inhibits an enzyme called **glucose-6-phosphate dehydrogenase (G6PD)** which puts glucose into storage.

 Less p53 means more glucose is available for the growth of cancer cells because there is unregulated glucose available for energy and cancerous cells use glucose faster than non-cancerous cells.

P53 is responsible for how cells divide making it very important in protecting the body from cancer. Mutations in p53 increase the risk of cancer. Up to 50% of reported cancer cases had mutations in the p53 genome.

More adrenaline means less p53 which means a greater risk of cancer. Chronic stress will cause chromosomal damage. You need to chill out and relax more. You will live longer.

Because your body is no longer repairing itself or has drastically slowed down the repair process you will age faster. You will not heal as easily. Your Telomeres (the protective caps on the ends of your DNA strands) begin to shorten short telomeres = short life long telomeres = long life. You will take longer to fight off infection. The organs constantly pumping out all these hormones also run the risk of burning out and malfunctioning.

PANIC ATTACKS

Post-traumatic stress disorder, obsessive compulsive disorder, Wilson's disease, pheochromocytoma (tumour of the adrenal gland), hypoglycaemia (low blood sugar), mitral valve prolapse and labyrinthitis (inner ear disturbances) can all manifest as panic attacks.

Vitamin B deficiency, a dramatic life change, death of a loved one, emotional trauma, life transition, stress, stimulants such as nicotine and caffeine (selective serotonin reuptake inhibitors) can also trigger panic attacks as can high blood levels of carbon dioxide. Withdrawal from drugs or alcohol can also cause a panic attack.

Your blood levels of stress hormones go up dramatically when you are having a panic attack. If you have never had a panic attack before it will seem as if you are having a heart attack and this will cause even greater distress. Panic attacks are best treated naturally rather than with drugs. Symptoms usually dissipate on their own, but will return at some point again if the root causes are not addressed. Make sure you are taking a good quality vitamin B-complex to minimize the risk of panic attacks.

TAKOTSUBO CARDIOMYOPATHY

This is also known as Broken Heart Syndrome or Stress-induced Cardiomyopathy. This affliction has all the symptoms of a heart attack although not as life threatening. The heart physically changes its shape to resemble a Japanese octopus trap called a takotsubo.

High levels of catecholamines, epinephrine (adrenaline), norepinephrine and dopamine brought on by intense emotional stress (like a traumatic medical diagnoses the death of a loved one natural disasters financial debt abuse etc. particularly when these things are unexpected but not limited only to the unexpected) grief fear resentment despair and anger cause the physical changes to occur.

It is a potentially life-threatening condition if left untreated. An estimated 1% of all heart attacks are related to stress cardiomyopathy. Treatment involves counselling and aspirin so his is not a drastic illness once it is diagnosed.

I include this condition here as an example of the physical changes that can occur to organs from prolonged exposure to stress and stress hormones.

Prolonged exposure to stress from whatever source **will** damage your health. It occurs on both a psychological and physical level under the influence of hormones.

Psychological changes will lead to physical changes if they are not addressed. The mind controls the body. Stress will affect your psychology (under the influence of erratic hormones) and your physical body (by inducing physical hormone-driven changes to your body). Make yourself aware of stressors and do your best to deal with them immediately.

Years of hard work in terms of diet and exercise can be undone within weeks from exposure to stress.

"For every minute you remain angry you give up sixty seconds of peace of mind." – Ralph Waldo Emerson

PERSONAL HEALTH

"Nine-tenths of our sickness can be prevented by right thinking plus right hygiene, nine-tenths of it!"

-Henry Miller

LOOKING AFTER YOUR PERSONAL HYGEINE

C-REACTIVE PROTEIN (CRP): The New England Journal of Medicine published an article that indicates that high **C-reactive protein (CRP)** levels are a stronger indicator of heart attacks and strokes than elevated cholesterol levels are.

C-reactive protein is measured to check the level of inflammation in the body and does not diagnose any specific illness. Infections, allergies, certain medications, insulin resistance, inflammatory conditions and obesity can raise CRP levels.

Being overweight will increase your CRP levels as bigger fat cells secrete **interleukin-6 (IL-6)** which stimulates the liver to produce CRP. Diet exercise and weight loss will help to lower CRP levels and with it the risk of heart attack stroke and diabetes.

Diets high in marine omega-3 fatty acids (EPA DPA and DHA) are very good at lowering CRP levels. Getting the correct balance of omega-3 and omega-6 fatty acids will boost this anti-inflammatory effect.

Animal research has suggested that a Paleo diet will lower blood pressure CRP levels and increase insulin sensitivity as opposed to a cereal based diet.[38]

Curcumin from turmeric, ginger, low-dose aspirin, Vitamin D, krill oil, omeg-3s, vitamin C and healthy diet and exercise will help lower CRP levels.

GUM DISEASE: causes bacterial by-products to enter the bloodstream via the gums and triggers the liver to make CRP which causes arterial inflammation and promotes blood clot formation. [39]

Tartar builds up on the gums and becomes saturated with bacteria. This becomes plaque which triggers body-wide inflammation. It also causes LDL cholesterol-related plaque to build up in the arteries. Some of the bacteria enter the bloodstream through the gums. You don't have to be a doctor to know that bacteria in the blood are not good!

Weight loss and oral hygiene dramatically reduce CRP levels so brush your teeth only floss the teeth you want to keep and make sure you use an antibacterial mouthwash!

Good oral health reduces the risk of heart disease diabetes and erectile dysfunction. For those with dentures you can still take care of your gums!

SINUSITIS: is another complication that needs to be addressed. The Para-nasal sinuses can become inflamed due to allergy infection or autoimmune disease.

Sinus inflammation can lead to a host of problems if untreated and the inflammation spreads. Inflammation of the sinuses creates similar issues as those brought on by gum disease i.e. high levels of CRP.

The causes are many ranging from viral to bacterial and even fungal infections. In type diabetes ketoacidosis is a cause of acute sinusitis.

If left untreated the complications of sinusitis include vertigo, abscesses, meningitis and infection of the brain by anaerobic bacteria. This can lead to personality changes hallucinations seizures coma and visual problems.

Consider using a NETI pot or a specifically designed squirt bottle to irrigate the sinuses with a specially formulated saline solution. These are all widely available at pharmacies. It should be used several times a day if you are experiencing sinus problems thereafter follow the manufacturer's directions for use. Drink lots of water to keep the mucus membranes hydrated. A last resort would be the use of antibiotics and corticosteroids.

There are psychological implications to not taking care of yourself. If you lose interest in taking care of yourself then you have lost interest in your health. That attitude needs to change if you want your health back.

GET ENOUGH SLEEP

Insufficient or poor quality sleep is associated with high blood glucose levels. It is unknown whether poor sleep makes diabetes worse or whether diabetes interferes with sleep but sleep deprivation and high blood glucose levels are connected.

The body repairs itself while we sleep so it makes sense to get at least eight hours of quality sleep each night along with adequate vitamins minerals and phytonutrients to assist in the repair process.

- Never watch television in the bedroom. It stimulates the mind too much and prevents the calming down period before sleep.
- Allow at least 2 hours after eating before going to sleep.
- Make sure that you get at least 8 hours of sleep per night.
- Use a sleep mask to ensure that your brain releases melatonin.
- Avoid high protein meals at night as certain proteins contain tryptophan which converts to serotonin. Serotonin will keep you awake.

Melatonin is only expressed in complete darkness and the best way to ensure this is to use a sleep mask to completely block out any and all ambient light and any light from electronic devices. Eat walnuts and cherries to boost melatonin levels.

It may seem a little silly and unnecessary, but the positive results are going to prove otherwise. The positive benefits of a healthy diet and exercise regime can be easily undone by insufficient or poor quality sleep.

STRESS REDUCTION

By now you should already be eating a healthy balanced diet with lots of vegetables nuts and berries and drinking pure water. You should also have stopped using stimulants like caffeine and nicotine and stopped using alcohol.

That means you are already doing something to combat stress! Diet has been shown to have a big impact on stress and how the body copes with it.Each of you will have interests or hobbies that you can adapt to help you better alleviate stress. These do **NOT** include sitting on the couch watching television all day or eating junk food!

Stress relief activities include:

- Meditation
- Exercise
- art
- Music
- Yoga
- Massage
- Tai chi
- Chewing gum –stimulates the vagus nerve and lowers salivary cortisol
- Pets – help to de-stress us
- Daydream - enjoy the view
- Laughter- endorphins relaxes blood vessels and increases blood flow

Meditation exercise art music yoga massage and **tai chi** are all proven to effectively counter stress. Get adequate sleep and try to avoid using sleeping medication to do this. Try using the delta wave soundtracks as a drug-free option to getting better sleep. Meditation is improved by listening to theta wave tracks.

Consider joining a class or gym so that you will be with like-minded people who can support you and whom you can support. Team environments have been shown to be more effective than solitary pursuits when it comes to motivation and the desire to improve yourself.

Exercise has been shown to promote a sense of wellbeing the goes beyond the physical effects. Regular exercise releases endorphins which counter the negative effects of cortisol and triggers the production of serotonin the feel-good hormone.

Chewing gum stimulates the **Vagus nerve.** This nerve conveys information about the organs to the central nervous system. Stimulation of this nerve reduces inflammation by preventing cytokine production. High levels of cytokines are connected with many diseases.

Vagus nerve stimulation is used as a treatment for drug or therapy resistant depression anxiety disorders migraines and tinnitus. Or you could buy a pack of sugar-free gum!

Studies have shown that **pets** can help lower stress and blood pressure levels. The Centres for Disease Control say that owning a pet may assist in lowering triglyceride and cholesterol levels. They increase self- esteem and psychological well-being and encourage physical activity. Pets are routinely used as therapy animals and many people recovering from heart attacks have benefitted from this.

Supplementing with an adrenal support supplement or adrenal rebuilder supplements may be necessary. Speak to a health professional that specialises in nutrition and ask them for supplements that will help with stress and adrenal fatigue.

Take some time out for relaxing and daydreaming. Personal time for introspection is never scheduled and many of us do not get time for ourselves the way we used to as kids. Find time for yourself. Make time for yourself.

There are many support organisations for stress out there. Your individual needs and circumstances will dictate where you go. Psychologists therapists priests or whoever you prefer are there to help you overcome problems that may be causing you stress.

BRAINWAVE THERAPY

Delta brainwaves oscillate at a frequency of between 0-4 hertz. They are associated with the deepest stage of sleep known as SWS or slow-wave sleep.

Delta waves stimulate the release of several hormones such as growth hormone releasing hormone (GHRH) and Prolactin (PRL). GHRH is released by the hypothalamus and stimulates the pituitary gland to release growth hormone (GH). Thyroid stimulating hormone (TSH) is decreased by delta waves so be careful if you any thyroid issues.

Disruptions in the delta wave sleep pattern have been linked to an increased risk of developing type 2 diabetes, possibly due to irregularities with the pituitary gland and growth hormone secretion. [40]

Other health issues with irregular delta wave patterns include Parkinson's, fibromyalgia, temporal lobe epilepsy, alcoholism, depression anxiety and OCD (obsessive-compulsive disorder).

Try listening to Delta wave tracks on your I-pod when going to sleep and Theta wave tracks when meditating. Theta waves are more 'inspirational' and "creative" in nature and are better suited to meditation.

You can do a Google search or a YouTube search for Delta wave tracks to download or listen to. Most are free to download and some even offer free brainwave generator software to download to create your own brainwave tracks.

DIABETES: CAN IT BE CURED?

We cannot solve our problems with the same thinking we used when we created them.
-Albert Einstein

THE "C' WORD

The "cure" for diabetes is the hot potato that nobody wants to hold. There is a huge amount of controversy over what a cure actually is or means. The dictionary definition of the word cure is:

Cure: kyʊər [ky*oor*] *Noun*
1. A means of healing or restoring to health; a remedy.
2. A method or course of remedial treatment as for disease.
3. Successful remedial treatment; restoration to health.
4. A means of correcting or relieving anything that is troublesome or detrimental: *to seek a cure for inflation.*

If you have removed all the criteria needed for the diagnoses of diabetes to be met and you are no longer taking any or require any medication for the treatment of diabetes does that not mean that you are cured?
If your pancreatic beta-cells have normalised and your organs are working as they should without the need for medication does that not constitute the right to call it a cure? If your HbA1c levels are consistently within the normal range is that also not enough evidence?

I have done this and yet I will always be labelled a diabetic because no precedent has yet been set.

There is a very adamant following of both medical practitioners and diabetes sufferers who refuse to acknowledge the possibility of a either cure for or reversal of diabetes. I call these people anti-curists!

 They appear to have fixated on being "incurable". The crux of their argument is that you are not cured; you are simply managing your diabetes with your diet, that you are a "controlled" diabetic. I disagree with this belief. Those who still take medication are "controlled".

If you refuse to change your diet and adopt a new lifestyle then you cannot expect positive change to occur. It does not mean that there is no cure just that there is no cure for you!

There is medical proof that diabetes is reversible yet people still refuse to accept this. Well, I refuse to accept the negativity of other people when it comes to my health. Choose your attitude!

Diabetes is a metabolic biological process that happens when certain conditions are met but it is a reversible metabolic biological process! There are claims made that you cannot cure diabetes because it means that you will never get it again even if you go back to eating pizza and donuts and drinking soda and fruit juice.

The ludicrousness of such a mind-set borders on insanity. Immunity to diabetes would be a wonderful thing but the biological possibility of such a thing escapes us right now (research is being conducted in this).

Diabetes has the potential to affect every living person on this planet and their cats, dogs, rats, mice and cows. The cause is almost always dietary related.

Recent scientific journals seem to indicate that endocrinologists are considering the possibility that diabetes is reversible based on test results from various sources. While many are willing to admit that it is possible to reverse diabetes, none are willing to put their names to acknowledging a cure yet for fear of ridicule from their peers.

There is more money to be made by treating sick people than there is to be made by educating them about diet and exercise. The financial stakes of continuously medicating a potential 25% of 7 billion people worldwide are astronomical. There is no money to be made by telling those people that a sensible diet and exercise will keep them off the medication.

Medication costs cents to make and dollars to purchase. 25% of 7 billion several times a day is a lot of dollars! Doctors will most likely never prescribe a diet before prescribing a course of medication. Doctors who do are perceived as quacks.

Many diabetic support associations and publications are heavily funded by drug companies and manufacturers of diabetic "equipment". Telling people there was a cure would be stepping on the toes of the people who pay the bills. The politics of finance are keeping diabetics in the dark and consequently diabetic.

A cured patient is lost revenue.

A study published in *Diabetologia* magazine proved that within one to eight weeks diabetes could be reversed through making dietary changes. It was once (and in some cases still is) believed that when pancreatic beta cells stop working they could never be resuscitated. This belief has been proven incorrect. This means that diabetes can be cured.

Diabetes is not just about keeping your blood sugar levels low either. In 2008 a US government study was conducted on 10 251 participants. The research experiment was done to test the effects on perfect blood sugar levels in diabetics but resulted in the deaths of more patients than that of a control group whose blood glucose levels fluctuated. The test used high risk patients and forced their blood sugar levels to near perfect scores but resulted in an unexpectedly high number of deaths from heart attacks.

Lowering their blood sugar to normal levels actually increased their risk of death! Perfect blood sugar levels will not save your life. [41]This does not mean that continuous high blood glucose levels are acceptable however. It implies that forcibly treating one aspect of diabetes means that you overlook many other aspects which will then step forward and cause damage. Treatment needs to be holistic and not specific. Look at the big picture not just the fine details.

Reversing diabetes is about lowering the intramyocellular fat by stimulating mitochondria to use up the fat so that insulin can get the glucose into those cells. It is about eating foods that will not spike your blood sugar. It is about making sure you get the correct supplements and nutrients. It is about enzymes fibre nutrients and much more. It is about using your body physically or losing it in pieces due to organ failure and amputation.

We consume foods that were not available to our ancestors hundreds of years ago in the vast concentrated quantities that are available today. Our lives may we busy and we may be stressed but we are not as physically active as our ancestors were. We have advanced technologically far beyond the ability of our biology to cope with these changes. The time has come to rediscover what the word "food" actually means.

The focus of manufacturers is on shelf life and profitability not nutritional value. We need to source food that is as close to its purest natural state as we can get it.

Our bodies have not yet caught up with the technology that has given us the "food" that sits on supermarket shelves. Can what we eat today even be called food?

Diet and exercise will take you out of the danger zone within weeks and months of starting them. This may lead you to become complacent and relaxed in terms of your health and what you eat. This is where things become dangerous. If you are feeling better there is more chance that you will slip into old habits. Be vigilant.

Years of bad habits will have caused damage to organs and systems that cannot be undone in a few weeks. You may be out of the high blood glucose danger zone but you still have a lot of repair work to do. This is going to take years of good diet and exercise to accomplish. Be strong! You need to adopt new lifestyle changes and create new good habits.

STEP UP

There is no easy way out of this! There is no magic pill that you can take that will make you non-diabetic. You are going to have to do this on your own. If you have the support of your family then it's a bonus.

I will paraphrase a quote by researcher Dr. Hardin Jones who at the time was speaking of cancer:

Diabetes is not a disease it is a survival mechanism.

Does that sound a little harsh? Perhaps but what that statement implies is that we are in some way responsible for causing our diabetes. If we continue eating garbage and not exercising it will kill us. If we prove ourselves unworthy of survival by eating non-food then we must face extinction. Only by changing how we do things and what we do can we hope to survive.

Insanity: doing the same thing over and over again and expecting different results.
-Albert Einstein

We need to reprogram ourselves and start doing things like eating healthy eating less exercising drinking pure filtered water developing a more relaxed approach to life and breaking our addiction to stress sweet things and stimulants.

Being overweight and sedentary are without a doubt the two most common factors leading to type 2 diabetes. Diabetics who have lost weight and begun exercising have shown remarkable improvements in their condition. Those who combined exercise and the resulting weight loss with specific diets have had complete reversal of their condition the same condition that was previously believed to be permanent and irreversible.

Reversing type 2 diabetes is about more than just making changes to diet and exercise. There is a strong psychological element to it too. Hormones control our moods and the organs that manufacture those hormones are negatively affected by diabetes. You will get emotional upheavals as your body detoxes and repairs. This will be very difficult but must be endured if you want to be cured. Your moods will stabilise eventually.

Cancer was once thought to be incurable and getting diagnosed with it was a death sentence. It is now beatable and there are many who survive cancer and they will tell you that the right mind frame is crucial in doing so.

If you truly want to reverse diabetes it is going to take effort dedication and commitment to accomplish. Diabetes will affect your moods emotions willpower and energy levels. You will not want to eat the foods nor do the exercises and you will get angry and frustrated.

These are all things to be aware of because if we are aware that they are going to happen we can take steps to overcome them.

WHAT SHOULD WE BE DOING?

We are trying to heal our bodies by supplying sufficient quantities of nutrient dense foods. We need vitamins, minerals and phytonutrients to repair damage and rebuild organs that have become worn out. We need fibre to remove waste and toxins. We need healthy fats to replace the bad ones. We need quality protein, in the right quantity, to rebuild tissue.

Most importantly, we need to stop consuming sugars and fructose in such consistently high amounts as frequently as we do.

We cannot do this with processed nutrient poor energy rich foods. We are trying to get our bodies to use up stored energy and not store more energy in the form of fat. This requires a dramatic change in our diets.

Human beings are concentrate-selective omnivores. This means that we require small amounts of nutrient dense food items from a wide selection of food sources for optimum health. We can survive on limited choices but it will eventually lead to ill health or death

Our present diets are high in energy but low in nutrients. This means that we survive from day to day in 2-steps – forward- 1- step- back manner. We get the basic nutrients to survive but not enough of the specific nutrients to repair our cells at an optimal level so that we thrive.

We aim to achieve this by diet and exercise and by removing "dead foods" from our diet and replacing them with "live foods" as I learned from DeWayne McCulley's book.

By adding physical exercise to our daily routine we will stimulate our metabolism to burn off stored fat. Exercise also benefits us in terms of improving circulation lowering cholesterol lowering blood pressure maintaining bone density and muscle strength improving joint flexibility and improving our moods by stimulating the release of endorphins.

By choosing the right type of proteins carbohydrates and fats with the correct ratio of proteins carbohydrates and fats we can repair tissue and have adequate energy without the highs and lows of erratic blood sugar. We will also minimise the amount of fat that gets stored.

Researchers at Monash University Medical School in Melbourne discovered that out of 55 patients with diabetes, 22 who had a stomach stapling procedure done were found to be no longer diabetic.[42] It appears as though calorie restricted diets and weight loss play a very major part in the reversal of diabetes but it is not as simple as that! Weight loss is a very important factor in reversing diabetes; there are many equally important factors that should not be overlooked. The correct types of calories are critically important too.

MY MISTAKE: What we eat is a very important part of the equation. I believed that I was doing the right thing by eating less of what I had always eaten and was surprised to find that my condition had gotten worse.

I had followed the guidelines given by the diabetes help associations thinking they would have a better understanding of the disease and knowledge on how to reverse it. They did not! It was all the same information I was already putting into practise with only negative results to show for my efforts.

I changed my diet again to include more low fat foods but there was still no improvement in my health. Low fat dairy and wheat products, high fibre anything, sugar free soda and fruit juice were added to my shopping cart. I added more fruit to my daily meals even canned fruits in light syrup.

The kind of foods I was eating was wrong. Low fat junk food is still junk food, it just has fewer calories! The nutritional components of my food were missing. I was not getting enough nutrients in my diet to heal my body. I was too focussed on the calorie content and not the nutrient density of my food. My foods were unintentionally pro-inflammatory. They were low fat, sugar free processed convenience foods. They had no real living nutrients left in them. I was also unaware of the toxicity of fructose.

I had completely missed the point of nutrition which is all about providing the body with the right building blocks to repair damage.

Enzymes, antioxidants, vitamins, minerals and phytochemicals are stripped from our foods during processing leaving behind only the basics like protein fat fibre and carbohydrates. This is why so many foods have labels advertising added vitamins and minerals to try and convince us that there is still some nutrition in them. There isn't!

There are not enough nutrients left in our food to repair damage anymore. All we get from our store bought convenience food is protein fat and energy most of which gets stored as fat when we do not burn it off. We are missing vital nutrition.

I researched until I found reports of cures and then re-searched those cures until I was certain they were not hoaxes. I was not happy with what I found because it went against the grain of conventional science and my lifestyle preferences. But I had to give it a try anyway.

I began eating more raw salads and started adding raw vegetable juices to my diet daily. I stopped drinking fruit juice and eating fruit which I had erroneously thought were good for me. I cut out grains and wheat and starches of any kind, gluten-free or not, unless they were sprouted grains. I drank more filtered water and took my supplements and multivitamins. I put in more effort at the gym. These changes paid off.

These are lifestyle changes as much as they are dietary changes but they were changes that I needed to make. As I learned what was good I would add it to my diet and as I learned what was bad I would remove it from my diet. I also added a substantial amount of raw food to my meal plan. I am neither a complete raw-foodist nor a vegetarian, but I assign these dietary aspects to a much larger part of my total diet than the cooked or carnivore aspects.

I started feeling better and made the decision to stop taking medication without consulting my doctor. This was serious decision to make but I was resolved to do it regardless of the possible negative consequences. I focussed on the positive consequences instead. My blood tests were coming back reading as if they were from a non-diabetic. There were no signs of diabetes in my blood work and I was not on any medication at all.

I know that I will never be able to stop the aging process that affects each and every single one of us until we finally run out of life. That was never my goal. I wanted to achieve a state of near perfect health and I believe that I am well on my way to doing that. The goal is to reverse illness and repair damage and restore the body to a level of health and low toxicity that we last had as kids.

HOW CAN I CURE MYSELF?

The only way I can see this happening is by eating more raw unprocessed organic foods. Raw foods will have more living components which would normally be destroyed by cooking. Cooking destroys a significant percentage of the protein in any food as well as all the enzymes and many other important nutrients making cooked food nowhere near as nutrient dense as raw food.

By eating more raw vegetables and drinking raw vegetable juice we ensure that we get enough fibre enzymes and nutrients. This puts less pressure on the digestive system and also less potential for allergy-related inflammatory responses from the immune system. This should allow the body to focus its limited resources on repairing the organs and systems affected by diabetes instead of putting out all the little fires.

If you intend eating animal protein then it must come from grass fed free range organic sources. It must not be farm-fed if at all possible. The wilder your meat is the healthier it is for you. This applies to any animal protein from eggs to animals to fish. Just make sure that you get your portion sizes right too much of a good thing is a bad thing.

Organic foods will have stronger defences against disease since they have not been treated with any chemical pesticides or growth hormones. This is good for our bodies since they are more nutrient dense even if they are less aesthetically pleasing. It also means that there is less potential for pesticide residues and growth hormones which the body will either store or process.

Garbage in garbage out!

Following a vegan diet (raw or cooked) for at least 30 days should, in most cases, reset the body to a pre-diabetic state. This gives you a firm starting point from which to work from. The more vegan and raw the diet is, the better the results will be.

Exercise is another important aspect of reversing and curing diabetes. Our bodies are designed to be physically active. Our present culture is so far removed from what our bodies are designed to do that it not surprising that we are suffering from so many metabolic diseases.

LET'S GET
STARTED

A journey of a thousand miles begins with a

Single step.

-Lao-tzu

WEIGHT LOSS

Getting your weight under control is one of the best ways to get your blood sugar and therefore your diabetes under control. There is a massive amount of evidence to support the claims that weight loss will assist in reversal of diabetes. We all know this. It needs to happen. Enough said!

Do not focus on taking the easy way out by trying diet supplements. The only effective way to do this is through exercise and a healthy diet plan.

Do not overthink weight loss and do not focus too much on weight loss. It needs to happen naturally and should not be forced. If you place too much emphasis on weight loss you can easily lose motivation if things do not move at the pace that you want them to.

You DO need to lose weight, but you must allow it to happen naturally, but stay focussed on the long term results and what you need to do to in order to achieve them.

EXERCISE

Exercise reduces stress and inhibits the release of the stress hormone cortisol. You also eat less when you are stressed. Exercise improves the Krebs Cycle (AKA Citric Acid Cycle or the Tricarboxyclic Acid Cycle) which is a series of chemical reactions that the body uses to generate energy by oxidizing acetate derived from carbohydrates, fats and proteins into carbon dioxide and water.

Exercise speeds up this cycle which detoxifies fructose and improves liver insulin sensitivity which means fructose gets used instead of stored. Research has shown that exercise lowers cholesterol and triglycerides and improves glucose tolerance particularly with resistance exercise.

AEROBIC EXERCISE: This is oxygen fuelled exercise. With adequate fuel and oxygen your muscle will not fatigue during exercise which is needed for long duration low intensity exercises like walking or jogging.

Aerobic exercise strengthens the lungs and heart and increases red blood cells which carry oxygen. It improves circulation and helps lower blood pressure. Aerobic exercise is also believed to improve mental health by reducing stress and depression. Let's not forget the fat burning benefits too.

Aerobic exercise is good for stimulating the circulatory system and removing toxins via sweat. It's one of the best ways to get oxygen into your system. The benefits of aerobic exercises are short lived so they need to be performed on a regular basis.

WEIGHT RESISTANCE EXERCISE: This refers to exercise in which the muscles are fuelled by things other than oxygen such as glucose. Weight /resistance training improves skeletal muscle insulin sensitivity (insulin works better in lean muscle) and thereby lowers blood sugar levels (the muscles use glucose for energy).

Anaerobic exercise also increases bone and tendon strength and has been shown to slow down osteoporosis in patients. Weight training will also help maintain muscle mass if you are on a calorie restricted diet which could otherwise cause muscle loss (in a state of low protein intake the body uses up its own protein for things it considers to be of greater importance a process called catabolism).

Weight training boosts the metabolic rate i.e. it speeds up the metabolism. Aerobic exercises will burn fat while you perform them but stops being of benefit when you finish.

Weight training increases your resting metabolic rate which means that you continue to burn fat (minimally) for several hours after you have finished exercising. The body needs to repair the muscle cells and in doing so it expends energy. Weight resistance exercise is absolutely a must if you want to burn fat.

WHICH TYPE OF EXERCISE?

Both types of exercise should make it onto your to-do list. They both have benefits and both types of exercise should be performed. Neither should be ignored in favour of the other. Do what you are capable of take it slowly one step at a time until you feel yourself getting fitter and leaner. Join a group or gym or see a personal trainer for a consultation to meet your specific needs.

Performing 20 minutes of exercise at least 6 times a week minimum is recommended. 2 hours per week out of the 168 per week is not an impossible task. One of the best motivators is joining a class or group. People tend to be more motivated and competitive in groups.

You need to exercise for your fitness level and for this reason I recommend joining a group or seeing a personal trainer. A professional advisor will be better able to assist you and prevent injury. They should also help motivate you to keep going.

IRISIN
Exercise stimulates the release of the hormone Irisin which turns white adipose fat (WAT) into brown adipose fat (BAT). Brown Adipose fat burns white adipose fat for energy.

Irisin improves glucose tolerance and raises insulin levels. BAT releases the hormone Thermogenin (UCP1) in response to cold which burns WAT to generate warmth resulting in weight loss. Swimming in cold water is one of the best forms of exercise for weight loss. The physical exercise will stimulate the release of Irisin. Irisin turns WAT into BAT. BAT is stimulated by cold into burning WAT for heat production.

Get swimming if you want to burn fat!

DIETARY APPROACHES TO CURING DIABETES

"Let food be thy medicine and medicine be thy food"

-Hippocrates

THE RAW VEGAN DIET

Following a raw vegan diet for 30 days has been shown to completely reverse the effects of diabetes to cure it in fact. If your condition has been poorly managed or you have been diabetic for many years it may take a little longer to undo the damage.

This is arguably the best approach to reversing diabetes but it is also the most difficult approach for most people. Of all the dietary approaches a raw vegan diet will have the most profound positive effect on your health but it is also the most difficult lifestyle for people to adjust to.

Dr. Gabriel Cousens is a registered medical doctor who has cured diabetics with a raw vegan dietary regimen. Following on his heels is Dr. Stefan Ripich and Jim Healthy who also advocate a mostly raw dietary approach to reversing diabetes. Both groups recommend supplements as a part of their programs.

The DVD *"Simply Raw: reversing diabetes in 30 days"* chronicles the story of 6 Americans with diabetes one of whom is a type 1diabetic. They are given a diet consisting entirely of raw vegan foods to eat. They are asked to give up meat, dairy, sugar, alcohol, nicotine, caffeine, soda, junk food, fast food, processed food packaged food and cooked food for 30 days. You do not have to live with diabetes. Following a strict diet for one month is a small price to pay to cure what was once called an incurable disease.

There are a growing number of excellent websites where raw foodies are happy to share their recipes and many blogs where people can chat and ask for support or assistance. Try to avoid the high fat recipes if you do start a raw vegan diet initially. A high fibre low fat and low protein diet is the recommended choice for diabetics who are trying to reverse their diabetes according to Dr. Cousens.

Omega-3s and omega-6s are taken in from nuts and seeds and not from oils. Virgin Olive oil is the only oil used and that is reserved mainly for salad dressings. Supplementing with fish or krill oil supplements is necessary however. Saturated fat from coconut flesh or virgin coconut oil is recommended in small amounts either in smoothies (fat shakes) or when making raw desserts. I personally took 2-3 tablespoons plain throughout the day allowing the coconut oil to dissolve under my tongue.

The focus is on raw vegetables with particular emphasis on leafy green vegetables. These are eaten as salads or pureed as soups or as green juices or green smoothies. According to raw food advocate and author, Victoria Boutenko, leafy green vegetables have the closest match to human dietary requirements for vitamins minerals and other nutrients.

CAUTION: You need to rotate your greens. All green vegetables contain small amounts of toxic alkaloids to prevent over-consumption and possible extinction of the plant. Each type of leafy green will have a different type of alkaloid present. Spinach has oxalic acid and bok choy has the myrosinase enzyme which causes hypothyroidism.

Eating too much of any one particular thing will cause a toxic build-up of whatever happens to be in that particular green. We need to focus on a broad selection of foods to obtain a broad selection of nutrients and to avoid toxic build-up from any one plant toxin.

IMPORTANT: this does not mean that leafy greens are toxic!

Consuming any one food item to excess will result in ill health no matter what that particular food item may be. In fact the very same toxins in smaller doses will have anti-cancer properties or anti-microbial properties.
Be sensible and rotate your greens. Eat as wide a variety of greens as you can.

As I have mentioned before human beings are concentrate selective omnivores. We need small amounts of food items from a wide selection in order to thrive. We get sick eating too much of the same thing, unlike ruminants.

Rotate your greens!

All vegetables have some form of toxin as a means of protecting its survival or continuation on the planet. Eat too much of it and you get sick and don't want to eat it again anytime soon. Cruciferous vegetables have goitrogens. Potatoes and tomatoes may contain solanine, and the list goes on. The point is small amounts of food from a wide variety of unprocessed organic sources will do you no harm. Eating from one source only is either obsessive or indulgent and will cause you harm.

It is advisable to have at least 7-9 different leafy greens that you can choose from and make sure that you rotate them when making green smoothies, juices soups or salads. Try kale, spinach, collard greens, romaine lettuce, Swiss chard, parsley, coriander leaf (cilantro), beet greens, dandelion greens, nettles, lambsquarters, micro greens, sunflower sprouts, arugula (rocket) and watercress.

There are many more you will need to experiment in order to find greens that suit your tastes. Most supermarkets sell Mesclun or baby salad greens. It is not difficult to get at least one decent leafy green vegetable salad per day is it?

Vegetable juices are allowed but not fruit juices because of their fructose content. Most root vegetables and some other vegetables do have small fructose content and in small amounts this is tolerable. If the juice is sweet it's probably because of the fructose. This just means that you should exercise moderation when making sweet vegetable juices such as carrot or beetroot juice and weigh the positive health benefits over the negatives.

Small amounts of fruit are added to smoothies on occasion for both palatability and enzyme content. Examples of this would be papaya (pawpaw), mango, kiwifruit, pineapple and young coconut meat. Fruit with high fibre content will slow down the absorption of fructose but fruit should nevertheless still be restricted.

A raw vegan diet will prevent the formation of AGEs which are linked to aging and disease and also prevent inflammatory responses from the immune system since there are no inflammatory compounds in a raw vegan diet (unless you have a food allergy to a particular food item).

Try a raw vegan diet for 25-30 days with blood tests done before during and after so that you and your doctor can see the difference. If you do not adjust your medication when on this diet you may run the risk of insulin shock occurring adjusts faster than anticipated so be aware of this possibility and inform your doctor or caregiver. You will need professional medical advice on how to adjust your medication.

The Raw Vegan Diet is not a calorie restricted diet. There is no limit to how much you can eat during your 3 regular daily meals. Make sure that you drink your 6-9 glasses of water per day along with any green juices or smoothies.

Your body will get all the necessary nutrients and fibre to repair and detox but you will still need to burn off stored energy i.e. fat. It should not dramatically spike your blood glucose levels but the body does react unpredictably in the first few days on a raw diet so expect the unexpected.

It will also not stimulate any inflammatory responses from the body. This is good in terms of using the immune systems resources for healing rather than fighting food allergies etc.as is the potential with cooked or processed foods. Many of us have allergies in varying degrees to foods that we eat every day. We never realise these allergies exist because we are never get tested for them. They negatively affect our health in the long term but are unnoticed in the present.

A raw vegan diet eliminates exposure to allergenic foods so that the body can focus its resources on healing rather than dealing with inflammatory responses. You will notice little things getting better as your diet progresses.

When you begin a raw food diet initially you can expect bad breath headaches tiredness and diarrhoea. This is normal. This is a detox diet. Your body is detoxing and some discomfort is to be expected. There are also some unexpected emotional responses that occur during a vegan diet changeover. This is possibly due to hormonal adjustments that your thyroid is making. You will find an improvement in your moods as time progresses so just stick it out you will get there.

You will require extreme self-discipline to attempt this diet as it is known to be one of the most challenging diets around. The food is usually the biggest hurdle to overcome. Some people stay raw vegans while others adopt a significantly healthier lifestyle than they had before. Adding raw vegetable juices and more raw foods to your diet daily will benefit you greatly if you choose not to go raw completely.

At present I am not a raw vegan but have adopted many of the principles of the lifestyle. I follow The Pareto Principle (the 80/20 principle) and try to follow an 80% raw 20% cooked diet. I also apply this to vegetables (80%) and animal protein (20%). These are my personal preferences. When you begin this diet it is advised that you follow a completely raw vegan diet for 30 days minimum. Regular blood tests should be done to track your progress until you are satisfied with the results.

www.YoungOnRaw.com

Mimi Kirk has written a raw un-cookbook called: *Live Raw: Raw Food Recipes for Good Health and Timeless Beauty,* which contains many incredible raw recipes to try. There is no lack of creativity or flavour in these recipes. It is a truly impressive recipe collection.

Enzymes in raw vegetables enzymes break down food assisting the immune system and perform the functions of metabolism. Lipase breaks down fat protease breaks down protein and amylase breaks down starch. These are just 3 enzymes out of thousands that we need to function optimally.

These enzymes are destroyed during cooking but not during juicing. If you use a high speed shredding juicer you must drink the juice immediately as the oxygenation produced by such juicers will affect the juice by oxidising it. Grinding juicers do not have the same problems and juice made by these juicers can be kept refrigerated for a day or so.

Cooking also raises the glycemic value of foods and it destroys vitamins and proteins. Most vegetables can be eaten raw and even some grains and pulses can be sprouted and eaten raw in this way. The biggest obstacle is our own mistaken belief that raw food will make us ill. This has got to change. Raw food is living, cooked food is dead.

If you do decide to try a raw vegan approach to reversing diabetes you need to have an exit plan. There must be a clearly defined start and finish to the diet. 30 days is the normal time frame and thereafter healthy cooked foods may be added to the diet in small amounts if desired.

A raw vegan diet is a complex and varied diet that does require a lot of work and preparation in order to meet the body's nutritional demands. You run the risk of deficiencies if you do not pay close attention to what you eat or do not take adequate supplements. You will need to check your iron and vitamin B12 levels regularly and supplement accordingly if needed.

Because a raw vegan diet is low in protein it is not advisable to exercise heavily during this period. Perform very light exercises such as yoga or walking but not aerobic or weight resistance exercises as these will place a demand for extra protein to repair muscle tissue. There is also potential to cause the down-regulation of thyroid hormones if the caloric input does not meet the energy output sufficiently. You can rectify this with the addition of coconut oil and avocados alongside the addition of high protein raw nuts and seeds.

Insufficient protein intake will lead to catabolism as the body diverts protein from other internal areas to repair muscle tissue. You may also become vitamin and mineral deficient as your body uses up nutrients and sweats out electrolytes.

A raw vegan approach is a very calm relaxed approach to reversing diabetes and there should be no physical or psychological stresses involved during the reversal process. If you do wish to exercise you will need to consult with a nutritionist who is familiar with your condition.

Electrolytes are easily replaced by drinking fresh coconut water and there are several raw vegan protein supplements available if you do have the energy for exercise. Check with your doctor or healthcare provider and ask them to assess your fitness level if you do want to start exercising while on a raw vegan diet.

Avoid fruit at all cost but consume as much raw vegetable juice and raw vegetable salads as you like paying particular attention to leafy green vegetables like kale spinach and silver beet (Swiss chard). You need at least 1Lb /450g of raw greens per day for optimal health. This can be in the form of a salad or a green smoothie or raw green juice.

Remember to rotate your greens to avoid toxic overload of any one particular vegetable and do not eat too much goitrogen rich cruciferous vegetables. Cabbage and broccoli may be superfoods but eating too much of them raw will cause havoc with your thyroid. Cooking denatures goitrogens so this might be considered as an option after the raw diet.

Successful healthy raw diets are incredibly varied and complex. Many people try a raw diet and become ill because they focus too much on too narrow a selection of vegetables. This is caused by toxicity from either phytochemical or vitamin build-up or nutritional deficiencies caused by not enough variety in the diet.

Consult a nutritionist and explain what you are trying to do so that they can give you advice and design a well-balanced raw meal plan. This should also include a comprehensive dietary supplement list. Be sure to tell them if you plan on exercising and at what level you plan to exercise at.

Make certain that you add Vitamin B12 and iron to the other supplements that you should also be taking.

VEGAN DIET

A vegan diet that includes both raw and cooked foods is an example of a lifestyle change that will reverse diabetes and keep it reversed. It should be a low fat diet and you should still keep fructose intake to an absolute minimum.

Vegans can fall prey to health issues just as easily as non-vegans if they do not pay attention to their diets. It is possible to be a vegan and have high cholesterol levels, for example.

Much of this can be attributed to lack of exercise, genetics and poor diet, even a vegan diet, if there is a lot of saturated fat and refined foods in the diet. Relying on processed and refined foods along with a sedentary lifestyle will cause sickness and disease.

A plant based vegan diet consists, ideally, of unprocessed, minimally refined wholefoods. There should not be any refined fats (cooking oils) or refined carbohydrates (sugars or syrups) in it, and remember to exercise.

There is plenty of evidence to support a vegan diet as a means of re-versing and even curing type 2 diabetes. Get started now, it does get easier.

Dr. Neal Barnard has written and spoken extensively on the benefits of a vegan diet. He has also proven the effectiveness of vegan diet in reversing type 2 diabetes.

A vegan diet does not have to be boring and it does not need to be exclusively raw. Some foods provide better nutrient absorption when cooked. Like the lycopene in tomatoes or the beta carotene in carrots. Some foods are only safe to eat when cooked, such as taro root for example.

A vegan diet that has cooked elements as well as raw elements will allow more flexibility and ease of use than an exclusively raw diet, but care should be taken not to fall into the convenience foods trap.

You should also make sure that you keep your diet diverse. Do not rely on French fries as your daily meal or eat vegan junk food options in the belief that they are healthy because of the vegan label attached to them.

Common sense is still required when choosing what you eat and relying on advertising or marketing to tell you what you can or cannot eat will only result in disappointment.

42nd president of the USA, Bill Clinton and many famous actors like Brad Pitt and Woody Harrelson are all standing in a long line of celebrities who have adopted a vegan diet.

A vegan diet, whether raw or regular, will show results within 30 days. Be sure to follow a low glycaemic diet and avoid fruit or fruit juice for the first 30 days

Whole fruit can be added after 30 days but fruit juices should still be avoided.

NOTES

INTERMEDIETE DIETARY PROTOCOLS

"A journey of a thousand miles begins with a single step"

-Lao-tzu

BEGINNING TO START

Many of us find it too difficult to jump in at the deep end and "just do it". This lack of conviction causes us to fail and become despondent and we soon quit, citing that "it doesn't work".

Well, it does work! But with this in mind, there are some intermediate-ate dietary options to follow that will make it easier to transition to a vegan or even raw vegan diet.

By taking baby steps we can slowly improve our health and adjust to new ways of eating and new foods to enjoy. A raw vegan or even a cooked vegan diet will make dramatic improvements in your health, but may be difficult for many to adopt overnight. Start slowly if you find it hard, but at least make a start!

Do not quit before you have even started. Take it slowly, but persevere and you will succeed. Work towards adding more vegetables to your diet and eliminating animal proteins and fats.

THE MEDITERRANEAN DIET

The Mediterranean diet does not consist of pasta dishes and artisan breads. These are popular misconceptions that seem to originate from television and movies.

It contains plenty of vegetables salads legumes olives olive oil and fish. There is a moderate consumption of red wine and red meat. Whole grains and nuts feature in this diet also. Pasta is an occasional food that is often seen on the table when large groups of people need to be fed.

Dr. Fedon Lindberg is a respected Norwegian endocrinologist who has written about how the Mediterranean Diet can reverse diabetes. The diet is low GI with a high vegetable intake. It recommends foods to be processed as little as possible if at all.

This diet is more lifestyle orientated than merely diet focussed. There has to be an element of physical activity involved for it to be successful. When ethnic groups are studied for their longevity their diet is usually the focal point but their physical activities never get as much attention.

The Mediterranean lifestyle is a physically active. It is a labour intensive agricultural lifestyle. Do not expect any miracles to happen just by following a diet; you will need to exercise too.

THE SLOW CARB DIET

This diet advocates a high protein low fat diet with lots of vegetables and legumes and the complete avoidance of any white starchy foods at all. Tim Ferriss made this diet famous in his book *"The Four Hour Body"*.

It is a fat loss diet that critics have called a cross between the Atkins diet and the Mediterranean diet. I have not found any claims to suggest that this diet will reverse or cure diabetes but the principles of the diet are sound. This is a diet for those unwilling to give up cooked food and meat and want to lose weight. You will need to exercise if you intend to follow this diet.

It has received international acclaim as a fat loss diet and may be worth looking at as a means to weight loss for diabetics. The cheat day could include virgin coconut oil and fatty foods like avocado and nuts rather than unhealthy candy, cupcakes and donuts as the "cheats". No sugar or fruit juices allowed ever!

This diet appears to be targeted at people who want to lose excess weight and get a little fitter at the same time. This is a high protein diet similar to the ketogenic diet and the paleo diet and you are going to need to exercise if you intend on following this diet.

I personally like the daily allowance of one glass of red wine. I justify it by saying that it is how I get my daily dose of resveratrol.

It's medicinal!

This is a good diet to try if you struggle to give up animal protein. It can be used as a transitional diet on your way to veganism.

On the following page is a list of the rules for the diet by Tim Ferriss.

The rules according to Tim Ferriss:

Rule #1: Avoid "white" starchy carbohydrates
anything that can be considered white. This means all bread pasta rice potatoes and grains. If you have to ask don't eat it.

Rule #2: Eat the same few meals over and over again.
Particularly for breakfast and lunch.

Rule #3: Eat a protein rich breakfast.
This should be done within 30 minutes of waking up in order to boost the metabolism

Rule #4: Don't drink calories.
Like alcohol or soda or juice. 1 glass of red wine per night for health and sanity is allowed.

Rule #5: Don't eat fruit.
(Fructose →glycerol phosphate →more bodyfat). Avocado and tomatoes are the exceptions to the fruit rule.

Rule #6: Eat as much:
eggs chicken grass-fed beef pork lentils black beans pinto beans spinach and mixed vegetables as you want.

Rule#7: Nominate 1 day per week as a cheat day.
This has a beneficial effect on the thyroid preventing it from becoming underactive. Be sensible in choosing cheat day foods.

DEFENDING THE CHEAT DAY:

A low calorie diet produces less T4 and T3 (thyroid hormones that regulate metabolic rate) so having a cheat day will ensure the production of these vitally important hormones. It will allow the thyroid to relax and not go into shutdown mode.

The exact same principle applies to leptin levels while on a low calorie diet (fasting and low calorie diets will lower leptin levels). A big caloric load will boost the metabolism by forcing the body out of adjusting to a low calorie mode.

For a diabetic to take a cheat day off their diet does not mean eating whatever the hell they want. It means choosing healthier options of treat foods.

This may mean that you have to make your own treats using fruits berries virgin coconut oil and nuts or avocado. Browse through the dessert sections of raw vegan un-cookbooks for some ideas.

This diet is very similar in concept as the one followed by DeWayne McCulley when he reversed his diabetes. It advocates the avoidance of any starchy carbohydrates and sugars including fruit juice and fruit itself dairy except for cottage cheese and grains and oats. You are advised to drink plenty of water and take supplements. Your produce both meat and vegetables should be sourced from organic sources wherever possible.

Both cooked foods and salads are allowed as are some fats. Meat is allowed since you are required to perform a reasonable amount of aerobic and anaerobic exercise.

This may not be the diet to reverse diabetes but it is a sound dietary approach to follow post diabetes if you are not going to go raw or vegan. Remember that meat is allowed only if you are exercising or you run the risk of high cholesterol levels and several other health issues surrounding high animal protein intake.

The slow carb diet focusses on protein and slow release carbohydrates. There is a reasonable amount of variation if you are creative but remember not to use any fruit juice (except avocado, tomato, lemons, limes and maybe grapefruit occasionally).

While I have not found any claims that it will cure diabetes it might be of benefit to those who do not wish to take on a very strict diet. It might also be an option for people who need a lifestyle diet to follow post-diabetes.

The principles of the diet are a mix of paleo and ketogenic and offer a bit more leeway for a busy modern lifestyle.

PALEO FOODS DIET

Consider doing some research on Paleo Foods and deciding how much of the principles of a Paleo foods diet you want to incorporate into your life. The basic principle is that our bodies were designed to consume unprocessed wholefoods such as wild leafy vegetables and roots, lean meats, fish and shellfish, eggs, nuts, berries and seasonal fruits eaten raw or baked / roasted without any additional fats or oils.

It excludes beans, grains, cereals and legumes, salt, sugar, dairy and processed foods and oils. Only fresh seasonal local foods are eaten but there are exceptions made for dried foods and frozen unprocessed foods. Foods may be cooked or eaten raw as long as no oil or salt is used in the process. In simple terms it is a high protein low carbohydrate organic diet with a few twists.

Gastroenterologist Walter L. Voegtlin published a book in 1975 arguing the validity of a Palaeolithic diet and its health benefits. After seeing the destruction caused by a "modern" diet on many of his patients he began to experiment with a simplified diet to cure them. He believed that farming and agriculture brought with them diseases of affluence. By limiting the types of foods we have access to we limit the amount and types of nutrients we get. He believed that we were hunter-gatherers and that our bodies had evolved to eating in that way.

A randomised trial involving 29 people with glucose intolerance and ischemic heart disease fed on a paleo diet showed greater improvements than compared to test subjects following the Mediterranean diet. Animal studies have seen greater insulin sensitivity lower C-reactive protein levels and lower blood pressure when fed a Paleo diet.

Another trial tested the results between a recommended diabetes diet and the Paleo diet. The Paleo diet accounted for lower values of HbA1c triacylglycerol diastolic blood pressure body mass index and waist circumference despite high animal protein intake. Glycaemic control and other cardiovascular factors were improved in both diets without any significant differences.

There are anecdotal reports from individuals who claim that the diet reversed their diabetes but I have not confirmed any of these. I would exercise caution as the diet does include large amounts of fruit and fats albeit unprocessed. You may need to customise this diet initially to suit the requirements of a diabetic. This means no fruit or sweet things like dates or raisins or any dried fruits would be allowed until you are no longer considered diabetic.

It may be a bit difficult for some to follow but the principles are sound and there are websites that have recipes and give advice. If you like sashimi (that's raw fish without rice), kokonda, escabeche, ceviche, carpaccio and jerky you may not find this diet too hard to swallow. A high protein diet may not be advisable for people with kidney damage, however.

There is a quite bit of controversy over the paleo diet since it does advocate a high animal protein and therefore saturated animal fat in however the principles of unrefined unprocessed natural wholefoods that are the basic concept behind the diet make it a sensible choice of diet.

I disagree with several points in the Paleo diet the avoidance of legumes is at the top of the list. The diet is a bit too extremist in terms of not acknowledging any positive benefits from eating foods not included in its hypothesis but this is a personal opinion. Those who follow a Paleo diet cite lectins as the reason behind these dietary exclusions.

LECTINS: lectins are anti-nutrients found in grains, legumes, dairy and plants from the nightshade family (potatoes, tomatoes, eggplants and capsicum peppers etc.) they are the plants' natural pesticide. Soybeans have one of the highest lectin contents of all legumes.

Lectins are sticky and work by binding to the villi of the small intestine. This prevents the villi from absorbing nutrients, vitamins, minerals and protein from ingested food. While lectins are known to destroy the epithelial cells of the intestines they are free to circulate in the body and can cause damage to the pancreas, the thyroid and collagen in the joints.

Lectins are connected to several food allergies inflammatory diseases and autoimmune diseases such as Crohn's disease, chronic fatigue syndrome, IBS, thyroiditis, colitis and rheumatoid arthritis.

Lectins are also believed to cause leptin resistance. Digestive enzymes break down some of the lectins but not all of it. Soaking sprouting and bacterial fermentation are pre-digestive techniques that help to remove lectins from food.

The Paleo diet seeks to eliminate any potential inflammatory compounds from the diet and therefore anything containing lectins.

Oats have been proven effective in lowering cholesterol levels and deliberately avoiding them while on a diet high in animal protein seems counterintuitive. If these grains and are sprouted and not cooked they have nutritional benefits that should not be ignored because of theoretical hypotheses. Olive oil and coconut oil also have benefits that would be unavailable to someone following the strict protocols of a Paleo diet.

We as a species need a wide selection of foods containing a wide selection of nutrients and excluding foods based only on theoretical hypotheses is narrow minded and potentially dangerous in the long term. By focussing only on a small selection of foods you lose out on the nutritional benefits to be had from a wider selection of foods.

Eating unprocessed organic and even wild vegetable foods means greater nutrient and fibre density. It also means that the foods will a different nutrient content to commercially farmed vegetables because of how and where they are grown. Eat a wide selection of wholefoods and wild foods that are unprocessed and unrefined.

Now that is my opinion and I am not a nutritionist or a medical doctor.

Dr. Robert H Lustig a well-respected endocrinologist gave a famous lecture called "Sugar: The Bitter Truth" available to watch on YouTube during which he said about the Pale Diet:

"…if you ate everything as it came out of the ground raw with no cooking you would cure diabetes on a dime takes about a week because you are getting that 100-300 grams of fibre..".

If someone of with his credentials is prepared to risk his credibility with a statement like that then this diet does warrant serious consideration.

THE KETOGENIC DIET
(LOW CARBHYDRATE KETOGENIC DIET (LCKD)

Studies have shown that a high fat high protein low carbohydrate diet can dramatically reduce HbA1c over several weeks and keeping daily blood glucose levels within acceptable ranges.[43] Insulin sensitivity also improved.

The ketogenic diet was initially used as a dietary treatment for epilepsy but research has shown that it is also of benefit to diabetics.[44]

On this diet only 20% of caloric intake should be from carbohydrates. The induction phase of the Atkins Diet is an example of a ketogenic diet.

Only 20g – 40g of carbohydrates are allowed per day. Three meals per day that contain high protein and moderate fat with a minimal amount of carbohydrates per meal sometimes no carbs at all if you have exceeded your daily allowance.

The Dr. Elliot Joslin Diabetic Diet from 1923 consisted of meats, poultry, game, fish, clear soups, gelatine, eggs, butter, olive oil, coffee, tea, with approximately 5% of energy from carbohydrates 20% from protein and 75% from fat. This was one of the earliest diabetic specific ketogenic diets.

The body switches from being a glucose fuelled machine to a ketone fuelled machine. Research has shown a dramatic decrease in HbA1c levels in patients following a ketogenic diet.

Animal studies using extremely diabetic mice found that a ketogenic diet reversed their diabetes *and* kidney disease caused by diabetes.[45]

The cyclic ketogenic diet (CKD) or carb-cycling diet as it is sometimes known is another version this diet. Several days of ketogenic diet are followed by several days of mostly complex carbohydrate. During this phase all fats and sugars, including fructose, are prohibited. For example Monday to Friday you follow a ketogenic diet and Saturday and Sunday you may eat carbohydrates.

The purpose of this phase is to refill the glycogen stores in the liver and muscles and also to combat the psychological aspects of carbohydrate cravings. There is also the issue of fibre and phytonutrient vitamin and mineral replenishing to consider. You may wish to consider combining a raw vegan diet with the CKD.

KETOSIS and DIABETIC KETOACIDODIS (DKA)

Ketosis :
Is essentially the body's way of using fat as fuel instead glucose. When the glycogen stores in the liver have run out the body then turns fat into ketones which are used as fuel. The body switches from using carbohydrate based energy to fat based energy sources.
The heart and kidneys prefer using ketones over glucose as energy. The brain can use ketones instead of glucose when it needs to.

Ketoacidosis:
 Occurs when there are too many ketones in the body. It is a metabolic state in which there are very high levels of ketones in the body. It occurs when there is a steady rise in blood glucose alongside a lack of insulin. It is more common in type 1 diabetics and alcoholics than in anyone else. Starvation diets can cause ketoacidosis in extreme cases. If you cannot produce insulin at all then you are at risk.

Diabetic ketoacidosis:
 Occurs when a diabetic becomes dehydrated and the body goes into a stress mode. Muscle tissue fat and liver cells are broken down and converted into glucose and fatty acids. The fatty acids are oxidized into ketones. The body cannibalises its own tissue for fuel. High blood glucose levels alongside a lack of insulin increases the risk of ketoacidosis.

If you have any issues with insulin production then you need to reconsider trying a ketogenic diet.

If you can smell nail polish remover or a fruity pear scent on your breath then you medical attention now! This is an indication of ketoacidosis.

De-stress and stay hydrated!

Ketosis- prone type 2 diabetes is an extremely rare condition that can affect someone on a ketogenic diet. It only happens when there is absolutely no insulin being produced at all. If you are unable to produce insulin at all then you should not attempt this diet without first consulting an endocrinologist.

There is anecdotal evidence of diabetics doing well on a ketogenic diet and not requiring any medications at all. Since there is a very limited carbohydrate intake there is not too much risk of high blood glucose levels.

You do need to be very careful about getting the balance right between too much fat and just enough fat. If you have high cholesterol levels it may be best to avoid this diet.

Consult a nutritionist or doctor to advise you whether this diet is suitable for you.

CALORIE RESTRICTED DIETS

Calorie restriction has been studied extensively. In both human and animal experimentation the results seem to agree living on a calorie restricted diet will help you live longer. Although it does have proven health benefits it is an extreme diet to follow. The positive results are hard to argue with though. This diet will activate the SIRT1 gene also called "the longevity gene" or "the skinny gene".

This is a brutal diet and only for those with titanium-strength willpower. If you believe that you are able to manage only 600 calories per day for a short period then give it a go.[46] It must be said that where the calories come from are just as important as how many calories there are. 100 calories from a double cheese pizza are not the same as 100 calories from a dressing-free garden salad.

While it has been proven that a calorie restricted diet will definitely reverse diabetes it is not a long term solution. Not many people are able to continue with a calorie restricted diet for extended periods without falling off the wagon. Use common sense and have a schedule or back-up plan for when to stop or if you should slip up.

Going on a calorie restricted diet for an extended period of time may cause your thyroid to slow down which causes other health issues to worry about. To counter this you may need to add coconut oil avocados and sea vegetables to your meals to avoid down-regulating thyroid hormone production so consulting a nutritionist beforehand is recommended if you want to go on any calorie restricted diet. Adequate supplementation will be necessary to avoid the risk of vitamin deficiencies

Consult a dietician if you want to try this diet strategy out. They will be better equipped to help you start and quit. They can also give you a menu of nutrient dense foods to choose from and how much you may consume each day.

On his website professor Roy Taylor has sample recipes used during clinical trials for reversing type 2 diabetes with a calorie restricted diet.

The web address below has the details of the study.

http://www.ncl.ac.uk/magres/assets/documents/StudyRecipes.pdf

These dietary guidelines can be down loaded and printed if desired. Definitely have a look at this site for an idea how to go about reversing diabetes through dietary means. This is a proven documented scientific method for reversing diabetes.

The diet included dietary supplements and low calorie protein shakes as a complement to a low calorie vegetable based meal plan which was followed for 8 weeks. This diet causes excess fat in the pancreas to disappear and the pancreas begins to function normally.

What you do afterwards will determine whether or not you remain diabetes free. Adopting a healthy diet and lifestyle that includes exercise and the avoidance of all sugars and fructose will ensure that you remain healthy.

This is a quick-fix dietary approach to reversing diabetes but it does not set the tone for what happens afterwards. Some of the test patients returned to their previous habits and became diabetic again.

Taking this into consideration you will need to have an exit strategy in place for after you have finished the diet.

You may want to consider adopting a Mediterranean diet or a slow carb diet or any of the other healthy diet lifestyle choices.

Going back to eating whatever you want is going to lead you back down the road to diabetes if you are not extremely careful.

ALTERNATE DAY CALORIE RESTRICTION (ADCR)[47]

This is another form of diet to consider. Research conducted on ADCR has confirmed physical and psychological health benefits for test subjects whether animal or human.

Within two weeks of starting an ADCR program improvements were seen starting in as little as two weeks in insulin resistance asthma seasonal allergies infectious diseases of viral, bacterial and fungal origin, bacterial tonsillitis, chronic sinusitis, periodontal disease, rheumatoid arthritis, osteoarthritis, Tourette's disease, Meniere's disease, cardiac arrhythmias and even menopause related hot flashes.

It is theorized that some conditions could be delayed prevented or improved including Alzheimer's, Parkinson's, multiple sclerosis and even some forms of stroke.

ADCR is to be used with a sensible low carb low GI/GL diet. On the days where food is consumed normally it should not be seen as an opportunity to gorge as this would negate the effects of the previous and next day's fasting. Think of it as one day of fasting and one day of eating a sensible healthy diet.

ADCR and regular fasting along with resveratrol supplementation will activate your SIRT1 gene which in layman's terms is the longevity gene. When the SIRT 1 gene is activated it produces proteins which protect the cells from degenerative diseases and premature aging. It is activated as a defence mechanism to protect cells. It curbs oxidative stress and inflammation.

SIRT 1 creates mitochondria in the cell which are like tiny powerplants that burn off intramyocellular fat that causes insulin resistance. SIRT 1 gene activators improve insulin sensitivity in adipose tissue liver and skeletal muscle. It also improves the glucose balance of the whole body.

It has been proven that calorie restriction can reverse diabetes and I believe that the SIRT 1 gene has a critical role to play in this. The health benefits gained by doing an occasional fast are well worth the minimal amount of discomfort caused by sensations of hunger.

CALORIE RESTRCITION AND HYPOTHYROIDISM

If you have hypothyroidism (slow or underactive thyroid) then going on a calorie restricted diet may damage your thyroid.

  Going on a calorie restricted diet for an extended period of time will cause T3 levels to drop by up to 50%. This means that you will slow down your metabolism even more and potentially damage your thyroid.

A study published in The American Journal of Physiology Endocrinology and Metabolism found that 25 days of calorie restriction reduced T3 production by 50 %. Other studies have found similar reductions in T3 levels in patients with insulin resistance and diabetes that go on calorie restricted diets. There are benefits but there are also risks. Make certain that you have a plan and stick to it. Consult with a nutritionist or doctor if you have any doubts.

A damaged thyroid leads to a host of other health issues such as bradycardia (low heart rate), osteoporosis (due to impaired calcium absorption) and other serious health issues such as high cholesterol levels.

If you have hypothyroidism you should not starve yourself. Make sure that you eat three meals per day, never skip meals and always eat breakfast.
 Leafy green vegetables and protein with every meal including breakfast will help to boost your metabolism too. There are vegan protein supplements available for those who want to stay vegetarian.

If you suffer from hypothyroidism you need to avoid all goitrogenic cruciferous vegetables such as cabbage, broccoli, cauliflower, turnips, kale, Brussels sprouts, mustard greens and peanuts. Most of these vegetables are highly nutritious superfoods and should not be eliminated from your diet completely. Cooking or light steaming will inactivate the goitrogenic compounds.

Avoid unfermented soya completely. Peanut butter and roasted peanuts are safe but raw peanuts should be avoided. Unfermented soy products, soybean oil, canola oil, raw peanuts, raw pine nuts and millet are all known goitrogens so eat in moderation only. If you have hypothyroid issues then avoid them completely.

Refined flour, sugar, caffeine, alcohol and hydrogenated or partially hydrogenated oils will place unnecessary stress on the thyroid yet another reason to eliminate them completely from the diet.

You should also make sure that your diet includes iodine, selenium,, zinc, copper, iron, vitamin A, B complex and vitamin C. Avocados and saturated fats such as those found in coconut oil stimulate thyroid function.

Sea vegetables contain iodine which assists in the production of thyroid hormones. Excessive consumption however can actually cause thyroid trouble due to excess iodine intake, so moderation is advised.

High stress levels have also been linked to hypothyroidism so keep your stress levels down. If you are uncertain about the condition of your thyroid you should ask your doctor to test your TSH (thyroid stimulating hormone) T3 and T4 levels. Make sure that you consult with a doctor or nutritionist before starting any diet.

There are many causes for hypothyroidism including diet and stress. Going on a calorie restricted diet if you have a thyroid issue is dangerous so be well advised before starting anything. Eating a healthy diet free from sugars and starches is a good starting point. Make sure that your diet is varied and that you do not focus on any one food item too much.

If you do decide to try a calorie restricted diet make sure that you have a clear starting and end finishing date scheduled and absolutely not more than 25 days in total. Make sure that you have your thyroid hormones' levels checked before and after the diet.

Make sure that avocado and coconut oil are added to your diet if you think you may have hypothyroidism as these have been shown to boost the metabolism. And keep your stress levels down!

THYROID HORMONES AND DIABETES

When you start a calorie restricted diet your metabolism slows down in an evolutionary response to hold onto fuel reserves which is bad. It does this by producing less thyroid hormones which are responsible for fat carbohydrate and protein metabolism. The thyroid down-regulates its production of hormones during periods of caloric restriction. It only makes sense for the body to hold onto reserve fuel when it believes it is near starvation just in case it does not get food any time soon.

By going on a binge once a week and only once a week after a calorie restricted diet you reboot the thyroid by letting it know that there is lots of food available so it can stop worrying and start producing more hormones. The thyroid can now up-regulate its production of hormones. A binge will theoretically reset or reboot the thyroid.

The 2 hormones behind all this are **Triiodothyronine (T3)** and **Thyroxine (T4)** which regulate the base metabolic rate and affect the growth and function of other body systems.

Thyroxine (T4) makes up 80% of the thyroid hormones in the body but is also the precursor to **Triiodothyronine (T3)** which makes up the other 20% of thyroid hormones. T3 is 300% more active than T4 and is the hormone responsible for increasing metabolism.

The pituitary gland in the brain is responsible for the production and release of **Thyroid Stimulating Hormone (TSH)**. The hypothalamus in the brain is responsible for producing **Thyroid Releasing Hormone (TRH)** which tells the pituitary gland to produce TSH.TSH stimulates the thyroid gland into producing T4 which leads to the production of T3.

When a certain level of thyroid hormones in the blood is reached the hypothalamus stops releasing TRH which stops the release of all the other thyroid hormones. When the thyroid hormones drop to a certain level the cycle starts up again. Viral infections stress and dietary deficiencies will affect this cycle negatively.

T4 is converted into T3 inside the body's cells. T4 does have other uses but its main function is as a prohormone i.e. creating T3. When enough T3 has been made any excess T4 will be turned into **Reverse T3 (RT3)**. It is a safety precaution performed in the liver and kidneys to prevent over-stimulating the metabolism and causing Hyperthyroidism from an excess of T3. Certain medications and chronic stress are causes for the production of RT3.

Excessive or unneeded production of RT3 will result in Hypothyroidism or a slow metabolism. High stress levels will produce high cortisol levels which will suppress the production of Thyroid Stimulating Hormone (TSH). This means that less T4 and consequently less T3 is being produced which leads to hypothyroidism.

Stress and the stress hormone Cortisol along with nutritional deficiencies of selenium iodine zinc and iron will affect the production of thyroid hormones. Calorie restriction will also have a negative impact on the production of thyroid hormones since the brain shuts down the entire metabolism to compensate for a starvation mode.

This is the reason for clearly defined start and finish times for a calorie restricted diet. Calorie restricted diets may have evidence backing them up for their life extension benefits but there are serious risks involved.

High blood sugar and low blood sugar can have a negative effect on the conversion of T4 to T3. A deficiency of iodine will result in a decreased production of T4 and T3 which causes the thyroid tissue to enlarge and becomes known as goitre.

Scientists at the University of Oklahoma Health Sciences Centre conducted research that showed that low levels of T3 correspond with blood sugar levels that are five times higher than normal levels. An injection of T3 dropped the blood glucose levels dramatically. T3 injections were briefly considered as a treatment option for diabetes. It regulates fat protein and carbohydrate metabolism.T3 directly boosts metabolism inside little cellular powerplants called mitochondria. This indicates a connection between diabetes and hypothyroidism. Low levels of T3 are also linked to high levels of LDL cholesterol and high triglycerides.

Mitochondria convert sugars and other stored organic molecules inside the cell to produce usable chemical energy or adenosine triphosphate (ATP).

There seems to be a higher than average number of type 2 diabetics with thyroid disorders often undiagnosed as symptoms of hyperthyroidism are mistaken for poor glucose control. Make sure you eat foods that contain **iodine** (shellfish, kelp, nori seaweed, kombu, garlic, lima beans, sesame seeds, spinach, kale, collard greens and Swiss chard), **zinc** (oysters, crab, chicken, turkey, cashews, almonds, peanuts and baked beans) and **selenium** (Brazil nuts, crab meat, salmon, halibut ,chicken) as these trace minerals are required for thyroid hormone(T3) production. Brazil nuts are by far the best dietary source of selenium. Selenium and Zinc are needed to turn T4 into T3.

It is vitally important to make sure that you get enough iodine in your diet since it is needed for the production of TSH and T4. Iodised table salt is being used less and less due to health concerns about too much sodium and we now run the risk of not getting enough iodine in our food. You can find iodine in seafood and sea vegetables like Kelp, Wakame and Kombu.

WAKAME

Wakame seaweed contains **fucoxanthin** which activates **UCP1** or **Thermogenin** (a fat burning protein) found only in the mitochondria of BAT (brown adipose tissue). It is a heat generating protein which may be of importance in weight loss.

Thermogenin is found in hibernating mammals and infants who do not have the same heat regulating mechanisms as adults. In simple terms it turns stored fat into heat rather than energy.

Wakame also contains the omega 3 fatty acid, eicosapentaenoic acid and high levels of calcium, niacin (vitamin B3), thiamine (vitamin B1) and iodine.

GLYCEMIC LOAD AND GLYEMIC INDEX

Glycemic load (GL) is the carbohydrate content in food portions. It uses the glycaemic index as a starting point and standard portion sizes for each different food item. GL tells us how much sugar will enter the bloodstream.

Glycemic Index (GI) tells if the food is a fast releasing carbohydrate or a slow releasing carbohydrate and how quickly a sugar will enter the bloodstream. **Glycaemic load (GL)** tells how much of the total food portion is from carbohydrates.

Together GI and GL will tell us what foods we can eat without worrying too much about high blood glucose levels, and what foods we can only eat small amounts of on occasion. It is wise to know both or at least have some understanding of the content of both in your food.

There are several websites dedicated to listing the glycemic indexes of various foods if you need to create a list of favourite foods and their glycemic indexes. Please take note of the differences in glycemic values between cooked and raw foods. Cooked foods will have a higher GI than raw foods.

A GI of 55 is low and a GL of 10 is low. It is necessary to know both the GI and the GL of a particular food to assess its suitability for your diet. Glucose sets the benchmark for Glycaemic Index at 100.

<u>GLYCAEMIC INDEX</u>		<u>GLYCAEMIC LOAD</u>	
LOW	- 0 - 55	LOW	- 0 - 10
MEDIUM	- 56 - 70	MEDIUM	- 11 – 19
HIGH	- 71 - 100	HIGH	- 20 and up-wards

According to Patrick Holford the rules are simple:

- 40 GL points per day to lose weight 60 points to maintain weight.
- Eat carbohydrates (not starchy carbs) with protein.
- Graze, do not Gorge! Eat several smaller meals per day rather than 2-3 large meals per day.
- Eat little but often and always eat breakfast. Breakfast must have protein and vegetable carbohydrates. A high protein meal no longer than 30 minutes after waking has been shown to have a beneficial effect on the metabolism.

Some research into the function of Leptin suggests that there should not be any snacking between meals.[5] The experts disagree so make your own decisions on whom to follow. You should allow yourself 2-6 hours between your last meal and bedtime. Your food needs adequate time to digest properly.

When you sleep your metabolism slows down. Your body concentrates its efforts on tissue repair while you are at rest. Going to sleep with a full stomach is the same as waking up with a bellyful of rotting food!

Digest before going to sleep so that you can have a good night's rest and so that your body is well stocked with nutrients to repair itself.

The GI and GL of any food can vary significantly depending on where it was grown. The reason for this will be determined by the soil type and nutrient content of the soil as well as growth boosters added to fertilisers etc. This is yet another reason to consider buying organic, locally grown produce.

I believe that a diet that focusses on GI/GL control is important and may be of some benefit for diabetics in controlling blood sugar but that attention must be given to what the food is and not just its GI. Low GI foods will help lower HbA1c levels over time.

---

[5] **The Leptin Diet**: How Fit Is Your Fat? (Take Charge), Byron J. Richards , ISBN:978-1-933927-28-2

Eating low GI rice crackers is not as nutritious as eating low GI salad greens. Leafy green vegetables are low GI and full of nutrients. They should be a large daily part of your diet.

It is very easy to lose sight of the big picture when you focus on the small details. Do not get caught up in counting calories when those calories are coming from nutrient poor sources. Calories are not the same as nutrients.

BASAL METABOLIC RATE

Your basal metabolic rate is the amount of energy needed to keep your body functioning while at rest. You need to find out what your BMR is in order to accurately assess what your daily caloric requirements are. You can do this online or through a dietician or nutritional therapist.

This will allow you to decide what amounts of fat carbohydrates and proteins you will need for the day. Exercise will raise your metabolic rate and consequently your caloric intake unless you are overweight and need to lose some weight in which case your caloric intake will be less.

If you chose not to exercise then you must eat less or you risk becoming overweight. More work = more food less work = less food. It is quite simple, really. Make sure that the calories you choose come from low GI, low fat and high fibre vegetable sources!

A CALORIE IS NOT JUST A CALORIE!

The caloric content of food is changed by how you process it. Raw celery burns more calories to process than it contains. Cooked celery does not. Cooked foods have a higher GI than raw foods and also a lower total nutritional value. Add significantly more raw foods to your diet for greater nutritional value.

100 calories from glucose is not the same as 100 calories from fructose. Every cell in the human body needs glucose for energy and unused glucose will be stored as glycogen whereas fructose is only stored as fat in the liver and will contribute towards insulin resistance and raise triglyceride levels.

They may both be 100 calories but how the body utilises them is completely different.

100g fructose - 279 calories   **100g sugar - 387** calories

fructose GI of 19-25   **Sugar GI of 65-80**

Taking this into consideration it would seem as if fructose is the logical choice to make but it clearly isn't.

Then there is the debate over cooked foods vs. raw foods. Cooked food might be easier to digest but unfortunately cooking will destroy most of the nutritional value and leave only energy value (GI) behind.

 Cooked food will have a higher GI than raw food and less nutritional content. Raw foods will have a higher fibre and enzyme content than cooked food but will not seem as palatable to many. It is best to process foods as little as possible for maximum nutritional value.

SIDE NOTE: Foods that have little or no carbohydrate will NOT have a GI value attached to them, e.g. protein. The ripeness of foods will also affect the GI value, as will the cooking method.
It is recommended that you keep your glycaemic load points below 50 per day for blood sugar control

INSULIN INDEX

Certain foods will raise your insulin levels. This is just as dangerous as high glucose levels, since insulin encourages fat storage. Animal proteins, baked goods made from white flour, fruits, potatoes and potato products and baked beans are some of the top offenders.

Avoid these foods if you want to avoid high insulin levels:

Foods made from white flour, foods made from potato, baked goods, baked beans, dairy products and candy are all insulinogenic so avoid them.

METABOLIC BOOSTERS

Certain foods are better at boosting metabolism than others. Below is a list of some of the foods reported to have benefit as metabolism boosters.

- **RAW NUTS:** like almonds, pecans, pistachios, walnuts and Brazil nuts. Make sure that they are RAW and not roasted or salted. Soak nuts to remove phytic acid.
- **CHILLI PEPPERS:** chillies contain capsaicin which has been shown to boost metabolism and encourage fat burning. Use chilli powder, chilli sauce (read the label carefully for any bad ingredients) and fresh or dried chillies liberally.
- **GINGER:** ginger is known to be good for many things, such as digestive ailments and motion sickness, but it also helps to speed up the metabolism. Use it as a tea, for salad dressings or stews. It is also available in capsule form for those not wanting to eat it.
- **CINNAMON:** cinnamon contains polyphenol polymers which act as insulin analogues. They mimic the action of insulin by getting glucose into cells. Since insulin leads to fat storage it means that less insulin equals less fat storage. Use cinnamon liberally on everything. It is also available as a capsule or an extract called cinnulin.
- **GREEN TEA:** polyphenols and caffeine in green tea stimulate thermogenesis and fat oxidation leading to weight loss. It is also available in capsule form.

PORTION SIZES AND CALORIC INTAKE

Energy from food is measured in calories or kilojoules. Carbohydrates, fats and proteins all have calorie content.

A rough guideline would be:

1g CARBOHYDRATE	**4 CALORIES**
1g PROTEIN	**4 CALORIES**
1g FAT	**9 CALORIES**
1g ALCOHOL	**7 CALORIES**

The average daily calorie intake is 2000 – 2700 calories depending on sex activity level and genetic factors.

Consult a nutritionist to help determine what your caloric needs are and then use this information to apply it to the types of foods that you wish to eat and what portion sizes are suitable for you. As you lose weight your caloric needs will change too.

Remember that raw foods will have a different GI to cooked foods and that the fibre content of raw food will burn calories in digestion.

You may already know that eating one candy bar requires several hours in a gym to work off. Most athletes are very strict with their caloric intake in terms of the quality and type of those calories. We need to start thinking this way too.

A low carbohydrate diet will mean lower blood glucose levels and if you are on medication for this you will need a doctor's advice on lowering your medication or coming off them entirely. This will mean lower HbA1c levels in the long term which is a good thing. But….

An increase in protein intake is potentially dangerous for someone with kidney disease so consult with your medical advisor before you start a new diet that is high in protein such as the Ketogenic diet Paleo diet or the Slow / Low carb diet.

If you are experiencing high stress levels then a diet high in animal protein will also cause high cholesterol levels (stress hormones are made from cholesterol) and excess cholesterol in the body is easily converted to bad LDL cholesterol.

If you are going to follow a low carbohydrate diet you will need to get your cellular fuel from somewhere other than glucose. Ketones are that other cellular fuel. The brain can meet up to 80% of its total energy requirements with ketones. This means a diet high in fat so again make sure you consult a doctor before trying it.

Certain tissues such as the lenses of the eyes red blood cells and the kidneys need glucose and ketones will not

suffice. For this reason the liver performs a process called
gluconeogenesis.

POST DIABETES

What happens after I have reversed my diabetes? Do I still have to continue with my diet? Can I go back to eating regular food?

ANSWER: your diabetes will come back for you if you call it. I cheat occasionally when in a social environment but my new life has come about because I have adopted a new lifestyle and taken on some new healthy habits in favour of the bad ones.

Your body will adjust and begin to require healthy food the way it did junk food. You may even experience nausea as I did when trying junk food for the first time after a long abstinence from it.

Your health needs to be made a priority, not your food preferences. Use common sense and remember what got you into trouble in the first place. It is for this reason that many would consider diabetes incurable. They feel that if they cannot eat whatever they want without fear of illness then there cannot be a cure. This is not the case. No-one on this planet is immune to the effects of poor nutrition.

Lifestyle changes need to be made and that will include breaking bad habits and addictions and adopting new healthy ones. It is not an easy journey but it is a necessary one if you want to live a life free from disease. The other option is pills and a slow death. Not for me thanks I'll pass.

Many of the things that I learned on my journey to health were things I did not want to hear and did not want to do. I listened and heard and I acted. I have not looked back since.

What most of the dietary protocols have in common is the avoidance of all sugars starches and processed foods and a focus on fresh, raw organic vegetables. The secret to health seems to be to avoid anything processed, concentrated or refined in any way. The more unprocessed and natural a product is, the healthier it will be.

These are lifestyle changes that need to be made and that does not mean for the short-term. You need to be in this for the long-term.

Too many diabetics complain that they have to stick to a diet for the rest of their lives in order to remain healthy. They choose instead to eat whatever they want and stay medicated. You cannot have your cake and eat!

You are responsible for deciding what to put inside your body, so if you make the wrong choices then **you** are ultimately responsible for **your** ill health. You need to own up to this fact and make the decision to change the bad habits into good, healthy ones.

 I would love to tell you that there is a diet of donuts and soda that will cure you, but there is no such thing. Welcome back to reality. Change your attitude towards *what* you eat and *how* you eat, and you *will* change your health for the better!

We all need to relearn what our food is all about. Our minds may very well be highly developed but our bodies are still in the Stone Age.

The food currently sitting on the supermarket shelves is unnatural to our bodies. Just because it does not make us ill in the short term does not exclude the fact that it does cause us to become diseased in the long term.

Eat more unprocessed and raw foods!

<h1 style="text-align:center">EAT MORE OF THESE FOODS</h1>

- **Raw vegetables,** especially **leafy green vegetables** like spinach, kale, silver beet/Swiss chard, collard greens, mustard greens, Asian leafy green vegetables, greens like broccoli, green beans, celery and watercress. Remember to rotate your greens and not focus exclusively on one type.

- **Fermented foods** like sauerkraut and kimchee), natto, tempeh and miso (just be cautious of high sodium content. These help populate beneficial intestinal flora and assist with digestion.

- Cabbage cauliflower radishes brussel sprouts and any other **cruciferous vegetables. Raw salad vegetables** like cos lettuce cucumber capsicum peppers bean sprouts tomatoes watercress chilli peppers and salad greens.

- **Sprouted vegetables.** Sprouted grains contain more proteins than carbohydrates due to enzymatic conversion of starches into protein.

- **Seeds** like Ground flax seed, hemp seed, sunflower seed, pumpkin seed and sesame seed. Many of these can be sprouted also.

- **Nuts** like walnut, Brazil, Almond, Pine nut, Peanut and Macadamia. Sprouted whole grains like Oats, Buckwheat, Pearl Barley, Rye brown, rice and Quinoa.

- Add **sea vegetables** like nori and kelp to your diet for the idodine that supports a healthy thyroid.

STOP EATING THESE FOODS

- **Starchy vegetables** such as baked and mashed potatoes chips/fries yams sweet potato / kumara and parsnips.
- **Sugar, Fruit yoghurts, Fruit juices** and Fruit canned in syrup, **Fruit drinks** containing added sugar Fizzy drinks containing sugar, **desserts** high in sugar, Iced cakes and pastries, filled **biscuits/cookies, doughnuts, Scones, crumpets, waffles ,Sweet pies,** etc.
- **Breakfast cereals** containing sugar or instant breakfast cereals.
- **White, Rice, Wheat, Corn,** and **rice pasta, Pizza White bread, baguettes, bagels, crackers, rice cakes**. Stay away from **anything white**.
- **Popcorn Crisps/chips** and other potato and corn-based snacks, Sweets/sugar candy and **chocolate bars/chocolate candy, High sugar jams/jelly, Table sugar, Ice cream,** anything containing **glucose syrup, High fructose corn syrup** or high levels of other **sugars**.
- **Fried foods spreads** and **dairy products.**
- Anything **processed, canned, vacuum sealed** or **preserved**.
- **Unfermented soy products.**
- **Processed or convenience foods.**

UNFERMENTED SOY PRODUCTS

Soy products are a vegetarian staple. Soya milk is widely available as a dairy milk substitute at the supermarkets. Soy protein and tofu are the vegetarian go-to protein sources.

The trouble is that unfermented soy products contain toxic phytochemicals. These anti-nutrients are called **phytates goitrogens** and **enzyme inhibitors**. These anti-nutrients act as the plants defence mechanism and immune system. They are designed to protect the plant from the sun, bacteria, viruses, fungi, bugs and us! They need to be removed before soya is safe to eat and the best way to do that is through fermentation.

PHYTATES: Phytates or phytic acid binds minerals like zinc copper iron magnesium and calcium. Deficiencies in these can lead to poor wound healing reproductive health nerve function issues and brain development problems. Fermentation breaks down phytates.

ENZYME INHIBITORS: Enzyme inhibitors in unfermented soy products interfere with the digestive enzymes amylase lipase and protease. This results in incomplete digestion of carbohydrates (amylase), fats (lipase) and proteins (protease). Intestinal bacteria now have to finish the job and this causes bloating discomfort and gas. If you have any digestive issues at all it is best that you avoid unfermented soy.

GOITROGENS: Goitrogens are substances which suppress the function of the thyroid gland by interfering with iodine uptake potentially causing enlargement of the thyroid gland (goitre). Goitrogens in soybeans interfere with proper thyroid function by inhibiting the conversion of T4 to T3 essentially slowing down the metabolism and causing hypothyroidism.

Isoflavones like genistein and daidzein found in soy have been shown to affect human estrogen receptors. Genistein does have medicinal benefits in terms of its anti-cancer abilities and anti-atherosclerosis properties so there are still some benefits amongst all the negatives. Caffeine in conjunction with iodine deficiencies may potentially cause thyroid cancer.

Care should be taken with eating cruciferous vegetables like cabbage, broccoli, kale etc. in large quantities as they are potentially goitrogenic. If you are juicing them you may well be getting too much of the potentially harmful phytochemicals in cruciferous vegetables. Juicing needs to be carefully considered as it is a way of getting concentrated amounts of nutrients into the body.

Other foods like peanuts, peaches, strawberries, radish and millet are also mildly goitrogenic and should not be eaten too frequently. Fermenting destroys the harmful compounds but leaves nutrients and good bacteria behind. Cooking will also inactivate these compounds.

Selenium iodine vitamin A vitamin D and folic acid are all beneficial for a healthy thyroid and many of us are not getting enough in our diets. Sea vegetables (kelp wakame etc.), avocados and the saturated fat from virgin coconut oil all have a beneficial effect on the thyroid.

VEGETABLES

When you go to the supermarket pay attention to what is at the entrance and around the outskirts as opposed to what is in the isles of the supermarket. You are being marketed psychologically targeted while shopping.

The vegetables are located near the entrance so that once you have chosen your healthy foods you no longer feel guilty about buying unhealthy treats snacks and convenience foods in the isles. This is a deliberate industrial psychology tool employed against you the consumer. This is not a conspiracy theory either it is standard practice in big retail supermarkets. Be aware of this and shop the outskirts of the store not the isles. Use a shopping list that you do not deviate from.

Leafy green vegetables brightly coloured vegetables cruciferous vegetables and salads should be made the cornerstone of your diet if you truly want to beat this disease! You should avoid starchy vegetables like potato and be cautious with vegetables like kumara sweet potato and pumpkin.

We should all be aiming for at least 1Lb / 500g each per day of raw leafy greens. That is a hefty amount which I am not able to do but still attempt. You can eat this as a salad or drink it as a green smoothie the choice is yours so long as it is raw. Victoria Boutenko is an author and raw food advocate who wrote "Green for Life". In the book she lists the nutritional components in leafy green vegetables. They are a near perfect match for the nutritional requirements for humans.

We need to concentrate on leafy greens and brightly coloured non-starchy vegetables. These are vegetables that have high nutritional value loaded with vitamins minerals fibre and phytonutrients. Consistent daily consumption of raw leafy green vegetables will help to lower your HbA1c levels over time.

Some vegetables to consider adding to your diet are; green beans (string beans), broccoli brussel sprouts, cabbage, spinach, kale, bok choy, pak choy, collard greens (bore-kale), Romaine lettuce, onions, garlic, ginger, chillies, chives, spring onions, celery, cucumber, capsicum, tomatoes, asparagus, bitter melon, okra, avocado and all salad leaves. All cruciferous vegetables are acceptable and help to improve liver function. Remember to rotate your vegetables and do not eat too much of any one thing too often.

Raw vegetables green smoothies and raw vegetable juices should account for at least 60-80% of your food intake. This may sound crazy but it is a proven method for reversing diabetes. The nutrient and fibre content of raw vegetables is unmatched by cooked food. Cooking destroys up to 50% of all the nutrients in vegetables and raises the GI.

You need to eat protein with carbohydrates to slow down the conversion to glucose so if you do eat something starchy it needs to be combined with protein and fibre. Lemon juice lime juice and vinegar have also been shown to slow down the absorption of carbohydrates so add a splash of balsamic vinegar or lemon juice to your vegetables or salad. Fibre does the same job if you are not a big fan of acidic foods.

MY MISTAKE: During my dietary intervention I was consuming more fruit and fruit juice under the mistaken belief that this was healthier. It was no surprise then that my test results were worse than ever. I was taking in more of the poison that caused my diabetes.

I believe that 1-2 pieces of fruit per week max are acceptable and even healthy but no more than that and definitely no fruit juice. (I make the exception for home-made green apple juice occasionally due to its high malic acid content and grapefruit juice which has benefits relating to glucose absorption) Notice that I used the word **occasionally**. Remember that fructose is poison!

When I switched to raw vegetable juices I noticed a distinct improvement in my health. Some foods appear to have more benefit for diabetics than others due to their specific phytonutrient content.

The long-term consumption of high GL foods is associated with type 2 diabetes and coronary heart disease. There is a greater risk of cancer with a high GI diet as cancer cells thrive on glucose.

Some foods may have a high GI but a low GL. Watermelon for example has a high GI (it is a fast releasing carbohydrate) of 72 but has a low GL (there is very little carbohydrate in 120g) of only 4 points. This means that while you may have been told to stay away from watermelon because of its high GI (which is true) you would have to eat large amounts of it to have a drastic effect on your blood glucose levels. A 120g serving of watermelon has only 6g of carbohydrate.

ENZYMES: Enzymes are protein molecules and ninety-eight of the 5000 known so far have been found in in the arteries. The there is a theory that over 100 000 enzymes are needed for the maintenance of a healthy body. They are crucial to healing digestion and metabolism.

Many fruits and vegetables and juices available on the supermarket shelves have had their enzymes destroyed by pasteurising or irradiation. These products will have a much longer shelf life but will now cause the pancreas to work harder to produce enzymes needed to replace the destroyed enzymes.

Cooking food also causes the destruction of enzymes and once again the pancreas will need to work harder to produce enzymes. Studies have shown that diets high in cooked foods cause the pancreas to enlarge over time. As the pancreas deteriorates over time it produces less enzymes and that leads to disease and illness. Eating more raw foods and drinking lots of raw vegetable juice daily will ensure that you get an adequate supply of vitamins minerals and enzymes. There will be less stress put on your pancreas and your body should heal faster.

FRUITS AND BERRIES

Fruits should generally be avoided as the fructose content should be avoided at all cost. Sour green apples are a rich source of malic acid which is a good anti-inflammatory and helps lower blood pressure so I chose to eat small amounts of them occasionally as a snack with nuts. I did occasionally add them to green juices to make them more palatable.

Some fruits are high in enzymes that are beneficial. Pineapple has bromelain a proteolytic enzyme (protein digesting) kiwifruit has actinidin (protease) and pawpaw (papaya) has papain (protease). Berries are a rich source of antioxidants to help fight the oxidative tissue damage that is present in diabetes and are good for breakfast smoothies.

The occasional piece of fruit in a smoothie or as a treat is acceptable as long as fruit is not a daily occurrence. Fruit is seasonal and our ancestors did not eat fruit daily. Our bodies are not able to cope with vast amounts of fruit on a daily basis all year long and most definitely not concentrated fruit juice. Fruit should always be consumed whole and not just as a juice. The fibre plays an important part in how the fructose is metabolised.

Berries like blueberries are a good source of anti-oxidants and other phytochemicals. Use them in smoothies or salads or as a snack but be cautious with dried berries as they are often treated with sugar and vegetable oil.

HEALTHY FATS

The human brain is 60% fat. We need fat! It is crucial to our survival but it has to be the right sort of fat I the right amount. Walnut oil macadamia nut oil flax (linseed) oil extra virgin olive oil ground flax seed and chia seeds are excellent sources of omega-3 and omega-6 polyunsaturated fats. These are not to be used in cooking however.

Nuts and seeds provide both protein and healthy fats rich in omega-3 and omega-6. Be cautious of having too much omega-6 fat as it can lead to inflammation if consumed in excess.

Add raw walnuts almonds sunflower seeds avocadoes and pumpkin seeds to your meals.

Food cooked in vegetable oil tends to be high in omega 6 fatty acid that along with the production of AGEs is why fried foods are so bad for us. Our modern diet also contains way too much omega-6 oils which are found in everything processed.

A good ratio of omega 6 to omega 3fatty acids is 2:1 and can be found occurring naturally in flaxseed oil. Our average today is 20:1 and has been used as an explanation for the meteoric rise in obesity diabetes and other serious health issues.

We need omega-6 fatty acids to be healthy but we are getting ten times the amount we actually need. Stop using cooking oils for cooking. Choose the best quality cold pressed oils you can afford and use them sparingly as dressings for salads.

ORGANIC FOOD

Organic foods whether animal vegetable or mineral should have as little added to them as possible either to make them grow bigger more in quantity or to prevent diseases and pests from bothering them. They should be as close to pure as possible and that means they will have blemishes so deal with it! Our food is intended to supply us with all the nutrition our bodies require and not just look good and have a longer shelf life.

Try shopping at local farmer's markets instead of buying imported foods that have been treated with gases to keep them from going bad during transport.

Organic locally grown foods will be fresher and more nutritious than imported foods that have been in storage for extended periods of time and will have a stronger natural resistance to diseases and infections since they are not reliant on pesticides and introduced chemicals. This translates into more naturally occurring phytochemicals which are of benefit to us.

The produce available at a local farmer's market or organic store will also teach you about seasonal foods i.e. what grows when and where it comes from in your particular region. Fruits and vegetables are seasonal or at least they used to be. We now eat fruits and vegetables out of season in quantities that our bodies have not yet evolved to cope with.

The human body has evolved over centuries to eat foods as they appear in season. We have changed that pattern. Is it any wonder that we now have so many metabolic diseases to plague us?

GMO FOODS

(Genetically Modified Organisms) are foods that have had their natural DNA forcibly changed to create a product that has different attributes to the original. This might be for a longer shelf life or to prevent spoilage or any number of reasons. On the outside this might seem like a good idea, but is it really?

When something has been genetically altered it will have a completely new DNA sequence we have corn with human DNA, tomatoes with moth DNA and goats with spider DNA to mention a few.. When you eat this food your body will not recognise it as a food that it is familiar with.

This will stimulate an inflammatory response from the immune system. You will not be poisoned by eating GMO foods because they are still food, but because of genetic engineering your body will perceive these foods as a threat and take action to protect itself.

You will still be getting proteins, vitamins, minerals, etc. as per normal, but you will now be getting a big dose of inflammation with your meal.

Stay away from GMO foods. The risks are not worth the cheaper price tags.

FIBRE

Fibre plays an important role in insulin sensitivity and weight management. It reduces the rate at which sugar is absorbed into the blood from the gut which means less sugar turns into fructose which means less fructose turns into fat. Fibre helps to make you feel "fuller" sooner by speeding up digestion and stimulating Peptide YY (PYY) which send a signal to the brain that you are now full. Fibre helps to supress insulin secretion by transporting fats to the colon where bacteroides turn the fats into short chain fatty acids which supress insulin secretion as opposed to long chain fatty acids which stimulate the secretion of insulin.

There are two types of fibre found in our foods:

Soluble Fibre or **prebiotic fibre** is any fibre which absorbs water to become a gelatinous viscous substance that is then fermented in the colon to produce bioactive by-products beneficial to the body. Sources of soluble fibre are beans peas lentils chia seeds oats rye barley broccoli carrots nuts and root vegetables.

Insoluble Fibre is not digested or fermented at all. It acts as a bulking medium and as a sort of internal broom to sweep out garbage. Sources of insoluble fibre are nuts flaxseeds wholegrains celery avocado green beans and the skins of tomatoes.

Soluble fibre binds to bile acids in the small intestine preventing them from entering the body and thereby lowering cholesterol. Soluble fibre reduces both the absorption of and response to sugar in the system.

Fibre helps to regulate our blood glucose levels and to remove toxins from our bodies. Our ancestors consumed as much as 100g of fibre per day. The daily average in our world is between 10-12 g per day. We should be aiming for a minimum of 50g per day.

There are fibre supplements available if you feel you are not getting enough in your diet. Adding a tablespoon of ground flaxseed/linseed to your meals is a good way to start. This will also add beneficial omega3s to your diet.

PHYTOCHEMICALS

Phytonutrients are substances taken from plants that are necessary for sustaining human life. This may be in the form of protein glucose or vitamins and minerals. Phytochemicals are non-nutritive compounds that protect plants in different ways. They appear to have health benefits for humans too. They are not considered essential nutrients but have more medicinal properties.

Both fall under the heading of Phytochemicals though and there are estimated to be more than 10 000 phytochemicals / phytonutrients in nature. So what are they and why do we need them?

Answer: They are naturally occurring biologically active molecules in plants fruits vegetables herbs etc. for example Salicin, the pain relieving anti-inflammatory phytochemical substance extracted from the willow tree, is synthetically reproduced to make aspirin!

Phytochemicals are basically plant medicines. They occur naturally in our raw unprocessed food. There are different classes of phytochemicals. They can be Carotenoids Flavonoids Phenols Lignans, Saponins, Sulfides, Terpenes and others.

They are involved in many different processes in our bodies. They prevent cell damage and cancer and lower cholesterol levels. They are precursors to many hormones in our bodies. We need them to repair detoxify and regulate various internal processes.

Here are a few that may be of interest to diabetics:

ALLICIN: Responsible for garlic-breath. More importantly it is a powerful antiviral antioxidant and antibacterial agent. It also improves circulation and claims have been made that it can lower blood pressure.

ANTHOCYANIDINS: These are a class of flavonoids responsible for the dark blue and purple colours of grapes berries red onions etc. They are found in fruits berries and vegetables. They are being studied for their benefit in the treatment of cancer diabetes inflammation bacterial infection aging and many more illnesses. You need more purple and blue foods in your diet if you are fighting inflammation. Red cabbage beetroot and blueberries are all rich in these flavonoids.

EPIGALLOCATECHIN (EGCG): this is a potent antioxidant found in green tea but not in black tea. It is believed to increase the metabolism and to promote fat burning.

Epigallocatechin improves glucose tolerance lowers triacylglycerol and increases insulin production. EGCG supplements have been used to treat diabetes in laboratory animals.[49] EGCG is available as a dietary supplement called **Teavigo®** or you could drink decaffeinated green tea. There are several decaffeinated green tea extracts available as dietary supplements.

PROANTHOCYANIDINS: Are another class of flavonoids with strong antioxidant properties. They are believed to help protect the body from internal and external toxins and to support normal metabolic functions stabilizing collagen and maintaining elastin. Collagen and elastin are needed to support organs blood vessels and muscle tissue.

Studies have shown the potential to prevent cardiovascular diseases by counteracting the negative effects of cholesterol on the heart and blood vessels.

You may have heard of the French Paradox where the French can consume high fat foods without any cholesterol or heart issues due to their consumption of proanthocyanidin-rich red wine. There is also evidence of anti-mutagenic properties. Pycnogenol and Resveratrol are examples of proanthocyanidins.

PHYTOSTEROLS: These are cholesterol-like steroid compounds similar to animal cholesterol but from plant origin. They have been proven to lower both cholesterol and triglycerides. Phytosterols compete with cholesterol for absorption in the intestinal tract thereby ensuring less cholesterol in the bloodstream.

Phytosterol supplementation is recommended for people taking statin drugs to lower their cholesterol rather than increasing the statin dosage. This is considered a safer option when considering the side effects of statin drugs.

Phytosterols are not made by the body so they need to come from our diet. Flaxseed Almonds Walnuts Pistachios Macadamia Wheat germ Peanuts Sunflower seeds Sesame seeds and olive oil are all good sources of Phytosterols. Phytosterols are available as a supplement if you choose to take them.

These are just a few examples of phytochemicals available in the foods we eat. There are too many to give as examples in one book. In order to benefit from Phytonutrients and Phytochemicals we need to get them from the food we eat or from supplements.

Make sure that you get plenty of fresh unprocessed vegetables and some whole fruits and berries. These will be the sources of many beneficial phytonutrients. Organic is best if you can afford it but the emphasis should be on raw fresh unprocessed vegetables.

All spices and herbs have beneficial phytochemicals so be certain to get whole unprocessed spices and not instant spice mixes loaded with fillers and "flavour enhancers". Learn to make your own spice mixes from whole spices and herbs or buy mixes from certified organic manufacturers.

Only drink fresh homemade vegetable juices. Occasionally you may want to make a smoothie with some whole fruit. Remember that it is the fibre in the fruit that slows down the metabolism of fructose and for this reason fibreless fruit juice is not an option. Store bought vegetable juices are essentially "dead" and no longer contain any living enzymes.

Try to drink at least one glass of vegetable juice daily and be sure to use many different vegetables so that there is no chance of overdosing on any particular substance. Variety is the key!

Store bought juices no longer have any real nutritional value left in them. The manufacturing processes used in there creation will have stripped any enzymes or nutrition from them. Stay away from store bought vegetable juices and make your own.

SUPPLEMENTS

Our food is becoming increasingly less nutrient dense. How our food is grown or raised where it was grown and what was used to affect its growth all have an impact on **our** nutrition.

Storage transportation and manufacture all destroy nutrients in our food so it is becoming critically important to supplement our diets with concentrated dietary supplements if we intend to avoid illness. Supplements need to become a part of our daily lives. A multivitamin and vitamin C should be taken should be taken twice a day regardless of how healthy you are.

Diabetics tend to have more specific supplementary requirements. The nature of the disease dictates the need for some supplements to protect against damage or to repair damage and other supplements because they are deficient. Below are a few dietary supplements that diabetics should consider taking. Always consult your doctor before you decide which and how much supplements you are going to take.

Most health professionals including doctors will tell you that it is a good idea to have some form of dietary supplement or vitamin complex.

Diabetics will have different supplement needs depending on how long they have been ill and how much damage has occurred to the various internal systems. This is something to discuss with your doctor or a nutritionist so that they can advise you on what to take and to avoid any interactions between supplements and medications.

Below is a list of the supplements a diabetic should consider taking.

SUPPLEMENT	AMOUNT PER DAY
Chromium (chromium polynicotinate)	600mcg split into 2-3 dosages
Omega-3 fish oil	1000 – 3000mg split into 2 dosages
Vitamin B-Complex	1 tablet 2x daily
Vitamin C	1000 – 2000mg split into 2-3 dosages
Multivitamin	1 tablet 2x daily
Coenzyme Q10	100mg 2x daily

SIDE NOTE: these are guidelines only! Always refer to the manufacturer's recommendations or your doctors recommendations when taking supplements!

Consult a nutritionist or other healthcare professional if you are on medication or are uncertain about what supplements may interact with each other.

ACETYL-L-CARNITINE: is an amino acid compound formed from the amino acids lysine and methionine. It helps to lower blood glucose levels and encourages the use of fat as a fuel source instead. It is also a potent anti-oxidant and has been used in the treatment of heart disease vascular disease and diabetic neuropathy.

It is used as a dietary supplement by people hoping to lose weight but has greater benefits than just weight loss. It is best taken at night since it stimulates the production of GH during sleep. It reduces leptin resistance in the brain and promotes normal glucose utilization by the brain. It helps to improve mood cognition stress resistance and combats depression.

ADRENAL AND GLANDULAR EXTRACTS: These are made from hormone-free porcine glands. Theses supplements contain the essential bioavailable building blocks necessary for repairing the adrenal and other endocrine glands that been put under stress and are close to burnout.

I include this as an extra supplement for consideration since not much thought is given to repairing the organs that have had to work so hard in diabetes, i.e. the adrenal glands, the kidneys, liver, pituitary, the pancreas, etc.

These supplements are used by people who have suffered from stress for many years and need to repair their adrenal glands which have become worn out.

Dosage varies according to manufacturer. I use Dr. Wilson's adrenal rebuilder but there are other brands available.

ALPHA-LIPOIC ACID (ALA): not to be confused with alpha linolenic acid Alpha-Lipoic Acid is a potent antioxidant and free-radical scavenger. It restores vitamin C and E and Glutathione which declines as we age. It is also responsible for eliminating toxic heavy metals from our systems. It is an insulin-mimetic with a very strong impact on glucose uptake. It allows GLUT-4 glucose transporters to let insulin into the cells. It reduces triglyceride production (fat storage) by allowing carbohydrates to be stored as glycogen rather than fat.

It is used to prevent organ dysfunction reduce endothelial dysfunction and improve albuminuria to treat or prevent cardiovascular disease, accelerate wound healing, reduce excess toxic iron and other heavy metals, to treat metabolic syndrome, improve or prevent age-related cognitive dysfunction, prevent or slow the progression of Alzheimer's Disease, prevent erectile dysfunction, prevent migraines, to treat multiple sclerosis, to treat oxidative stress , to reduce inflammation, treat peripheral artery disease and much more.

If you have any form of metabolic disease you need to take ALA.   400-900 mg per day is a recommended. ALA has absolutely no toxicity to humans and there are no daily requirements listed.

ASPIRIN: While not technically a supplement aspirin should still be a part of daily supplement regimes. 75mg-100mg per day is recommended. Aspirin has an antiplatelet effect by inhibiting the production of thromboxane which binds platelets together to create a patch over damaged walls of blood vessels. If the platelet patch becomes too large it causes a blockage which causes a stroke. This makes aspirin a necessary supplement for people at risk of heart attack or stroke.

Overuse of aspirin causes gastrointestinal bleeding which can lead to iron deficiency so do not overmedicate.

BITTER MELON EXTRACTRACT: Bitter melon contains an insulin-like plant protein called Polypeptide-p (a kind of plant insulin) which will help to lower blood glucose and HbA1c levels.

L-CARNOSINE: reduces the negative effects of excess adrenaline on the kidneys and helps reduce leptin resistance. It is also thought to help prevent Telomere shortening which causes aging heart attacks and other age-related illnesses.

CINNAMON: Cinnamon and the cinnamon extract called cinnulin have been proven to lower fasting blood glucose levels quite dramatically. Cinnamon has insulin-like properties which should help to lower blood glucose and HbA1c levels.it is high in antioxidants, vitamins and minerals that diabetics tend to be deficient in.it activates enzymes that in turn stimulate receptors in cells to respond better to insulin. It also inhibits the enzymes that cause insulin resistance. Take ½ to 1 teaspoon of cinnamon per day with food. It is available in capsule form too.

CINNULIN: Cinnulin is a water soluble extract of cinnamomum burmannii. Cinnulin has been used as a supplement to treat diabetes obesity metabolic disorders and blood clotting disorders. It has potent antibacterial properties and is believed to help improve memory. Cinnulin's beneficial effect on the metabolism also accounts for weight loss lower cholesterol and lower blood pressure. 500mg of cinnulin is the recommended dose.

CISSUS QUADRANGULARIS: Is a relatively unknown herb in the western world. It is used to treat bone fractures obesity heart disease diabetes high cholesterol stomach upset asthma and joint pain in Asia and Africa. Reports from people using it have been positive in its benefit for lowering triglycerides and in weight loss.

It has been used to treat obesity diabetes heart disease metabolic syndrome high cholesterol and strangely bone fractures. There also appears to be an anabolic element to using cissus quadrangularis and it is completely safe to use. Tests have shown antioxidant, anti-inflammatory and analgesic properties. It appears to have an effect against malaria too.

There is no daily limit set for the dosage but 2g 30 minutes before a meal seems to aid in weight loss. Do not exceed 7g per day total dosage.

CHROMIUM: AKA **Glucose Tolerance Factor (GTF)**
An essential trace mineral that assists with the metabolism of protein, fats and carbohydrates[50]. Research has shown that if you are diabetic or pre-diabetic you will most likely have a chromium deficiency.

It appears to both regulate and improve the action of insulin. Supplementation improves insulin efficiency in people with high blood sugar.[51] It has a normalising effect on insulin in people with low blood sugar essentially it has an overall blood sugar stabilising effect. Whenever you eat High GI foods your body depletes its chromium stores to process the glucose that is metabolised. This is made worse when you take into account the fact that most of the chromium is removed from our food during processing.

The two most important symptoms of a chromium deficiency are: decreased glucose tolerance and impaired glucose metabolism. Sound familiar?

Chromium works better than metformin but without any of the side effects. It improves insulin sensitivity supports normal carbohydrate metabolism and fat management; it begins to work faster and lowers blood glucose levels faster than metformin.

Do not take chromium with antacids as they reduce the amount of chromium your body absorbs. Chromium lowers blood glucose levels so if you are taking medication that does this you run the risk of having a hypo. Your medication needs to be adjusted or even stopped by your doctor to counter this. Chromium is an essential trace mineral metformin is not![52]

Brewer's yeast is an excellent food source for chromium if you do not wish to use supplements. A diabetic needs around 600mcg. Per day split into 2-3 doses. This is over

10 times the amount for a non-diabetic. Once you are no longer insulin resistant the dose can come down. A post-diabetes maintenance dose of 50mcg per day is normal. Chromium polynicotinate appears to be the safest and best form of chromium supplement.

CLA (CONJUGATED LINOLEI ACID): helps to reduce body fat by shifting the focus away from fat storage improves GH (growth hormone) function and is thought to help treat cancer diabetes and atherosclerosis.

COENZYME Q10: AKA Ubiquinone or ubidecarenone (because of its ubiquitous (widespread) distribution throughout the body is an oil-soluble vitamin-like substance. It generates energy in the form of ATP Adenosine Triphosphate which transports chemical energy within the cells.

Diabetics seem to have significantly lower levels of CoQ10 than healthy individuals. It is a powerful anti-oxidant that protects vitamin E which is the major anti-oxidant in cell membranes and blood cholesterol. It is used in the treatment of several heart diseases including congestive heart failure angina and heart arrhythmia. It significantly reduces high blood pressure and helps in healing from gum diseases.

Diabetics and people suffering from heart disease are known to be very deficient in this nutrient and statin drugs used to lower cholesterol interfere with the body's natural CoQ10 production. Low levels of CoQ10 have also been linked to Parkinson's disease. Age and exercise lower CoQ10 levels so if you are older or are exercising you will need to supplement withCoQ10.

Although it can be ingested from the diet in trace amounts this process requires vitamins and minerals and seventeen metabolic steps to accomplish so supplementing is essential. The effects are not instantaneous and may take up to eight weeks to be noticed.

CoQ10 has been used in the treatment of heart disease gum disease high blood pressure Parkinson's disease and diabetes[53] with positive results. It stimulates the UCP3 system which allows cells to get rid of excess saturated fat.

FULVIC ACID: this organic acid makes cell membranes more permeable and increases mineral uptake into the cells. It also removes toxic heavy metals from the system. Add it to raw vegetable juices to increase mineral availability.

GABA (GAMMA-AMINOBUTYRIC ACID): Gamma-Amino Butyric acid (GABA) is an amino acid that acts as a neurotransmitter in the central nervous system. It inhibits nerve transmission in the brain. It is a natural tranquilizer and anti-epileptic that calms nervous excitability. Researchers discovered that if they injected type 1 diabetes mice with GABA it reversed the disease.

It worked in the pancreas to regenerate insulin-producing beta cells and it acted on the immune system to stop the destruction of those cells. It cured the disease and prevented it from recurring. So not only does it calm your nerves it also helps to regenerate pancreatic beta cells. Not bad for a health store supplement. This supplement definitely deserves consideration.

GYMNEMA SYLVESTRE: Gymnema sylvestre(AKA the sugar destroyer) is an herb that grows in South-east Asia where it is used to treat diabetes, rheumatic arthritis, stomach ailments, constipation, water retention, liver disease, gout and for weight management.

It supports healthy glucose metabolism controlling insulin release and activity and healthy pancreatic function. Gymnema sylvestre contains compounds known as gymnemic acids and tritepenoid saponins and gymnemasins which support healthy blood sugar levels. The leaves have antibacterial compounds. Anti-allergic antiviral lipid lowering and other effects are also reported. Animal research indicates potential to maintain healthy cholesterol and triglyceride levels.

IRON: iron is troublesome but essential mineral. Too much is just as bad as too little. Vegans and vegetarians need to keep a close watch on their iron intake to make sure that they get enough. Iron combines with proteins to form haemoglobin in red blood cells and is essential in carrying oxygen from the lungs to cells farther away that are locked in tissue and muscle.

Iron deficiency is the most common cause of anemia and leaves people feeling tired lethargic short of breath dizzy and also causes heart palpitations and an inability to focus. Untreated iron deficiency can lead to organ failure.

Beans lentils Peas potatoes broccoli asparagus mint parsley lemon grass collard greens beetroot greens bok choy turnip greens morel mushrooms sundried tomatoes watercress and spinach dates raisins and turmeric are all high in iron.

Coffee tea soda grape juice and wine inhibit the uptake of iron. Vitamin C assists in the uptake of iron so foods rich in vitamin C should be paired with foods rich in iron for better absorption. If in doubt consult a doctor or nutritionist to recommend a supplement or dietary solution.

MAGNESIUM: Diabetics tend to have low magnesium levels which are easily overcome with supplementation. There is evidence to suggest that magnesium deficiency is connected to insulin resistance. Magnesium supplementation has improved insulin production in elderly type 2 diabetic patients. Magnesium supplentation may also help prevent diabetes-induced damage to the eyes in type 1 diabetics. It is important for cardiovascular health nerve and muscle functions and may help treat migraines. Overuse of magnesium can cause diarrhea.

MULTIVITAMINS: get a good multivitamin from a reputable company. They will usually advise taking 2 per day in separate doses. We need take multivitamins as a precaution a backup to ensure we are getting a broad spectrum of vitamins and minerals in our daily lives. Vitamin deficiencies are a contributing factor behind many illnesses.

If you drastically change your diet you may also inadvertently change your vitamin intake. Taking a supplement will ensure that you get everything you need in the right quantities. Remember to always check with a healthcare provider or nutritionist before taking supplements to ensure that it is safe for you to do so.

MILK THISTLE: has been used for thousands of years in Europe and Asia as treatment for both diabetes and kidney complaints. It contains Silibinin which protects pancreatic beta cells from IAPP cytotoxicity. Follow the manufacturer's directions.

NARINGENIN: This is a type of flavone and contains vitamin P and citrin and it's found in abundant quantities in grapefruit. It is a potent antioxidant and anti-inflammatory. It boosts the immune system and speeds up carbohydrate metabolism by acting as insulin mimic. It helps get the glucose into the cells. It also reduces ulcer formation and slows down oestrogen production by interfering with the chemical reactions that create oestrogen.

PYRUVATE: Mitochondria in your cells use pyruvic acid to convert nutrients into energy. Pyruvate supplementation is believed to increase energy levels and boost the metabolic rate. Studies have shown that pyruvate combined with exercise and good diet is an effective weight loss tool. It is also an excellent mood stabilizer.

RESVERATROL[54]: is a protective compound produced by red grapes and a few other plants. It exhibits anticancer anti-inflammatory anti-viral and cardiovascular supportive properties. Resveratrol has also been shown to lower blood glucose and blood lipid levels.

It reduces the "stickiness" of blood platelets meaning less possibility clumping together and causing a blockage keeping blood vessels open and flexible. Inside each cell there are microscopic mitochondria. These are responsible for turning fat inside the cell into energy. Diabetics appear to have too few mitochondria to burn up the intramyocellular fats.

Pyruvate supplements are thought to improve mitochondrial functions. Resveratrol supplementation increases SIRT 1 activity which in turn increases mitochondria. There is less SIRT 1 found in cells with insulin resistance and increasing SIRT 1 levels will increase insulin sensitivity. SIRT 1 is also known as the Longevity Gene.

VANADIUM[55]: Vanadium is a trace mineral that mimics insulin by driving glucose and amino acids into muscle but it appears to be more beneficial to the liver than muscle tissue in terms of its glucose lowering ability. CAUTION: If you have very high triglycerides you may not want to supplement with vanadium as it has been known to raise triglyceride levels in overweight and obese people.

There is evidence support a reduction in fasting blood glucose of up to 20% with vanadium supplementation. Type 1diabetics will require less insulin. Vanadium should not be taken consistently for an extended period of time as there may be a possibility of toxic overuse. 25mg doses twice a day with food is the normal dosage.

As with most supplements a sensible routine with breaks in-between cycles is advised. Consult a nutritionist for advice.

VINPOCETINE[56]A relatively new supplement, vinpocetine, is a semi-synthetic extract of the lesser periwinkle plant (vinca minor). It is reported to have anti-oxidant and cerebral blood-flow enhancing and neuroprotective benefits. It does this by increasing blood circulation in the brain.

It is believed to inhibit an enzyme called phosphodiesterase preventing damage to brain cells and increasing the brains use of oxygen. It is used in Eastern Europe and Japan to treat cerebrovascular disease and age related impairment.

It is a vasodilator nootropic and a potent anti-inflammatory used in the treatment of Parkinson's and Alzheimer's disease. There do not appear to be any side effects or drug interaction related to vinpocetine supplementation however it should be used with caution by people on blood-thinning medication or who have low blood pressure.

VITAMIN C: Vitamin C is the star among vitamins. Entire books are written about this vitamin alone. Take up to 100mg per day divided into 2-4 separate doses.

VITAMIN B12: Also known as Cobalamin. There are two forms of B12; Cyanocobalamin and Methylcobalamin. The body must convert Cyanocobalamin into Methylcobalamin so take that into account when shopping for supplements.

If you decide to follow a vegan diet then you will need to supplement with vitamin b12. A deficiency in B12 can cause anaemia and nervous system damage and elevated levels of homocysteine which cause a host of unpleasant illnesses including heart disease if left untreated.

If you are eating plenty of leafy greens then your folate intake should reduce the homocysteine levels but you may still need to supplement with additional B12.

VITAMIN D: plays a role in immunity and the formation of blood cells. It is necessary for adequate blood levels of insulin. Vitamin D specific receptors are found in the pancreas (where insulin is made) and it has been suggested that vitamin supplementation may assist in insulin production and secretion. There are statistics that suggest between 70-80% of all people are deficient in VitaminD3.

MY MISTAKE: I was taking higher than normal doses of some supplements and at some point started to feel unwell.

I adjusted my supplement intake by cutting back to normal recommended levels and that cleared things up.

At some point you are not going to need high doses of supplements so you need to check in with your doctor or healthcare provider to adjust your dosages. Everyone needs to take supplements no matter how healthy they may be. Our food is simply not delivering the goods anymore. We all need to take supplements if we intend to remain illness-free.

I believe that supplements can be taken on a roster so that the body does not become "immune" to them. It also helps prevent toxicity or bad interactions between supplements when you are taking several. Always consult with a professional medical advisor before taking supplements.

CAUTION: Supplementing with vitamins and minerals is becoming more important now than ever before but more is not necessarily better.

In 2004 studies reported that seemingly harmless Vitamin E supplements could in fact increase your risk of stroke. Taking 400IU or more of Vitamin E would dramatically raise the potential for having a stroke. This was increased even more if combined with something as simple as aspirin. Be cautious with your supplements. Consult with a nutritional expert or your doctor if you can or use lower dosages if unsure about combining with other medications.

A good quality multivitamin from a reputable brand will usually recommend 2-3 pills split up over the course of a day rather than one massive dose all at once. If at any point in time you start to feel unwell you should immediately consult with your medical professional and tell them exactly what supplements you are taking and what dosages. Health is not an exact science and adjustments will need to be made.

VEGETABLES OF INTEREST

APARAGUS: binds with bile acid which causes the liver needs to use more bad LDL cholesterol to make more bile. This means less LDL in your liver and bloodstream which is good. Lightly steamed asparagus appears do this better than raw asparagus.

AVOCADO: Rich in heart-friendly monounsaturated fats that lower bad LDL cholesterol and triglycerides and raise good HDL levels. Avocado is high in fat so try to limit the amount you eat and only eat fresh avocado not the processed guacamole stuff in the chilled foods section of the supermarket. It contains phytosterols including beta-sitosterol, stigmasterol and campesterol, carotenoid antioxidants including lutein, neoxanthin, beta-carotene and alpha-carotene, other (non-carotenoid) antioxidants including flavonoids like epicatechin, vitamins C and E and the minerals manganese, selenium and zinc and omega-3 fatty acids in the form of alpha-linolenic acid.

BLUEBERRIES: are high in anthocyanins, proanthocyanidins, resveratrol and flavonols. Research has shown consumption of blueberries to lower cholesterol and total blood lipids assist in maintaining normal blood pressure levels alleviate symptoms of depression and enhance memory and learning in older people.

Eat them with a handful of nuts as a snack and use frozen berries out of season for smoothies and sugar-free compote or coulis or as an addition to a homemade vegetable juice drink. Puree them with mixed frozen berries and pour into ice-lolly containers as healthy treats or dessert options.

BROCCOLI: this superfood is an excellent anti-oxidant and anti-inflammatory and a potent detox agent. Lightly steamed broccoli is exceptionally good at lowering cholesterol. Lutein and zeaxanthin found in broccoli are needed for good eye health.

BRUSSELS SPROUTS: glucosinolates found in Brussels sprouts offer protection against cancer. The fibre in them helps to lower cholesterol. Flavonoid antioxidants like isorhamnetin quercitin and kaempferol are found in Brussels sprouts as well as antioxidants like caffeic acid and ferulic acid

CABBAGE: red cabbage contains anthocyanins which are potent anti-oxidants. Savoy cabbage contains sinigrin which is being researched ion cancer prevention. Whichever colour or type of cabbage you prefer all are useful in achieving better health.

CAUTION: All cruciferous vegetables (cabbage, brussel sprouts, kale, broccoli, bok choy, mustard greens, turnips, arugula (rocket), collard greens etc. contain glucosinolates which in high doses are goitrogens that affect the production of thyroid hormones particularly people with iodine deficiency.

On the other hand glucosinolates have potent anti-cancer properties and contain enzymes and antioxidants that prevent the formation of several cancers. In sub-toxic amounts glucosinolates do more harm than good so caution is advised in eating too much of a good thing. Cabbage juice is pretty foul stuff; trust me I've been there.

Use caution and common sense if you are eating lots of cruciferous vegetables and make sure that you get enough iodine in your diet to counter this.

CHERRIES: anthocyanins in cherries act like anti-inflammatory agents by blocking the actions of cycloxygenase-1 and 2 enzymes. Cherries have potential to protect against chronic pain from ailments such as gou,t arthritis and fibromyalgia (painful muscle condition).

They are also rich in the anti-oxidant melatonin which has the ability to cross the blood-brain barrier easily and produces soothing effects on the brain neurons calming down nervous system irritability which helps relieve neurosis insomnia and headache conditions. You will also get a good night's sleep. It is a fruit so be careful of eating too much.

COS / ROMAINE LETTUCE: this lettuce is the most nutrient dense of all the lettuce family. It is rich in vitamins fibre and phytonutrients. It should be a regular addition to your meals. Use the leaves as wraps or as regular salad leaves.

FIGS: particularly dried figs contain chlorogenic acid that is believed to help lower and control blood glucose levels in type 2 diabetes. Dried figs are rich in B-complex vitamins such as niacin pyridoxine folate and pantothenic acid. These vitamins function as co-factors for metabolism of carbohydrates proteins and fats.

Dried figs are excellent sources of minerals like calcium, copper, potassium, manganese, iron, selenium and zinc. 100 g of dried figs contain 640 mg of potassium, 162 mg of calcium and 2.03 mg of iron. Potassium is an important component of cell and body fluids that helps controlling heart rate and blood pressure. Copper and Iron are needed for red blood cell formation and cellular oxidation.

Try and stay away from dried fruit as much as possible due to the high fructose content but an occasional treat for the sake of nutritional content may be beneficial. As long as you eat small amounts of whole fruit you will benefit from the fibre and other nutrients.

GRAPEFRUIT: Many of you have been told not to drink grapefruit juice because it interferes with your medication. It does so do not drink it if you are still on medication as it enhances some medicines and reduces the effectiveness of other medicines.

Naringenin is a type of flavonoid and is the predominant flavone in grapefruit. It is an anti-oxidant, free radical scavenger, anti-inflammatory, carbohydrate metabolism booster and immune system modulator. It reduces hepatitis C virus cell production and lowers blood and liver LDL levels. It has also been shown to reduce oxidative damage to DNA.

Naringenin in grapefruit juice opens up receptors in the muscles to allow blood glucose to enter and be used as a fuel rather than be stored as fat. You have a window of 1hour after eating to drink grapefruit juice and do some light exercise like squats to benefit from this.

GREEN BEANS: these beans are a source of carotenoids like lutein, beta-carotene, violaxanthin and neoxanthin and flavonoids like quercetin, kaemferol, catechins, epicate-chins and procyanidins. They are a source of vitamins A, C, K, B1, B2, B3 and B6. They are high in fibre and con-tain several essential minerals.

The high content of flavonoids and carotenoids in green beans will help to reduce the inflammation that is so com-mon in type 2 diabetes. Green bean juice is said to help lower blood glucose and whole raw green beans are be-lieved to help lower cholesterol. Add them to raw salads or juice them.

OLIVES: Olives and olive oil are rich in anti-oxidants and phenolics (plant substances that make blood less likely to clot) as well as heart-healthy monounsaturated fats that lower Bad LDL cholesterol and raise good HDL cholesterol.

ONION: There is evidence to show that sulphur compounds in onion can lower blood levels of cholesterol and triglycerides and also improve cell membrane function in red blood cells as well as improving bone density. Quercetin is a powerful flavonoid anti-oxidant found in onions that prevents the oxidation fatty acids inside the body.

SHIITAKE MUSHROOMS: Contain Lentinan[57] a beta-glucan, anti-tumour polysaccharide which is approved for use in Japan as an actual pharmaceutical drug for cancer treatment[58]. It also boosts the immune system. Another extract Eritadenine[59] has been shown to have dramatic cholesterol lowering effects. Better start adding these mushrooms to everything!

SPINACH: is rich in vitamins minerals phytonutrients and flavonoids which all provide antioxidant protection. It is one of the most nutrient dense foods available to us providing nutrition and protection against cancer oxidative stress inflammation and cardiovascular problems.

Spinach contains oxalates which inhibit calcium absorption but this is only an issue if you drink spinach juice several times a day. Eating spinach daily is fine and will not affect you at all. You will need concentrated amounts in large quantities for there to be any negative effect. Kidney stones are created from calcium oxalate so if you have any kidney issues you should use caution with spinach juice and minimise your intake other oxalate rich greens. Aside from that spinach should be a staple food in your vegetable pantry

TOMATOES: rich in Lycopene tomato is known for its cancer fighting ability and to prevent the formation of LDL cholesterol. 25mg of lycopene per day equates roughly to ½ cup of home-made tomato sauce.

NUTS

When selecting nuts, make sure that you choose raw nuts and not the salted roasted-in-vegetable-oil supermarket snack nuts. These are high in fat and sodium and have no nutritional value left in them except for fat content and minimal protein. These are high in omega-6 fats and will cause an imbalance in your omega fatty acid levels if you eat too much of them.

Some raw nuts like almonds may be soaked and sprouted to remove toxins in the skin and increase the protein and enzyme levels and the digestibility of the nuts.

ALMONDS: research has shown that eating almonds with a meal will lower the glycaemic index of the meal. Almonds contain B complex, Vitamin E, Folic acid, magnesium, potassium, calcium, phosphorous and selenium. They are high I protein fibre and antioxidants. The biotin in almonds helps to metabolise sugar and fat into usable energy.

Soak almonds in several changes of water to remove toxins in the skin. They can be added to smoothies or salads or eaten plain as a snack.

BRAZIL NUTS: are rich in mono-unsaturated fatty acids (MUFA) like palmitoleic acid and oleic acid that helps to lower LDL or "bad cholesterol" and increase HDL or "good cholesterol" in the blood. Just 4-6 Brazil nuts per day will provide you with your daily selenium requirement which helps protect against coronary artery disease cancer and liver cirrhosis.

WALNUTS: these nuts are an excellent source of omega 3 fatty acids. Research has shown that small amounts of walnuts consumed daily will reduce total cholesterol in diabetics. Add them to salads or eat as a snack.

SEEDS

Seeds are important sources ofomega-6 polyunsaturated fats. We need these types of fats to remain healthy but we get far too much up to 20 times the amount that we actually need simply by using cooking oils and eating foods that have been fried or had vegetable oil added to them.

We need to ditch the cooking oils and start eating more seeds to ensure a more balanced intake of omega-6 fatty acids. Seeds will provide protein fibre nutrients *and* omega-6 polyunsaturated fatty acids in the right amounts and not just concentrated amounts of these fats the way that using cooking oils will.

BUCKWHEAT: Not actually a grain at all but rather a plant fruit seed. It is also gluten free. It is rich in flavonoids like Rutin and phytonutrients. Rutin, a glucoside, strengthens capillary walls and reduces haemorrhaging in people with High Blood pressure and it increases microcirculation.

Buckwheat contains abundant quantities of D-Chiro-Inositol (DCI) which is an important secondary messenger in Insulin Signal Transduction. Diabetics tend to be deficient in of D-Chiro-Inositol (DCI). Research done on DCI has shown it to lower blood pressure increase insulin sensitivity and improve glucose disposal.

Buckwheat is 18% protein with a high concentration of all the essential amino acids in particular Lysine, Threonine and Tryptophan. It also contains iron, zinc and selenium. Diets high in in buckwheat have been linked to reduced risks of high cholesterol and high blood pressure. It is high in magnesium which is known to relax blood vessels and increase blood flow. There is research to show that phytonutrients in buckwheat may have a blood glucose lowering effect when it is made a regular part of the diet.

Buckwheat seed may be sprouted and added to salads or used as a substitute for rice. You can sprout buckwheat and dehydrate it to use as a breakfast cereal with oat or almond milk.

Although people with coeliac disease or gluten allergies can safely eat buckwheat there is a small percentage of the population who are fatally allergic to buckwheat. Check to make sure you have no allergies! Your doctor can perform an allergy test if you are uncertain.

CHIA: Chia is high in omega-3 fatty acids particularly α-linolenic acid (ALA). It is also a good source of anti-oxidants amino acids and essential minerals like phosphorous manganese calcium and potassium. The seeds may be sprouted and used in salads or sprinkled onto food included in baked goods or used in smoothies.

Cinnamic acids in chia seeds help to prevent omega-3 fatty acids from oxidising. Chia makes thick mucilage in water absorbing up to 30x its weight in water and helps to clean and detoxify the intestines as well as leaving you feeling "fuller" making it perfect for smoothies and puddings.

FLAXSEED / LINSEED: High in fibre protein micronutrients and essential fatty acids. Flaxseed is the richest source of Omega-3 fatty acids known to us. If you want to prevent Heart disease Hypertension and Inflammation then flaxseed needs to be a daily inclusion in your diet.

Flax seed boosts the immune system and helps to decrease platelet stickiness thereby reducing the risk of heart attack and stroke. Flaxseed is a rich source of Lignans, a type of phytoestrogen, help protect against cancer (particularly hormone related cancers). There are 800x more lignans in flax than any other plant source.

Flax helps to lower cholesterol and stabilises blood sugar levels. Oklahoma State University found that 38g of flaxseed per day can reduce LDL (bad) cholesterol by 14.7% and total cholesterol by 6.9%.

Ground flaxseed provided the best nutritional benefit but needs to be kept refrigerated as it will go rancid sooner than whole seeds. Grind your own flaxseed in a coffee mill or blender in small amounts and store in the fridge. Use it in smoothies sprinkled over foods or in sauces.

QUINOA: pronounced keen-wah. This superfood is a rich source of the essential amino acid lysine and is also a good source of dietary fibre, calcium, phosphorous and iron. Quinoa has a high protein content of 12-18% with a balanced set of amino acids which make it a complete protein.

The seeds may be sown to grow the plant whose leaves are suitable to use as a vegetable. Use quinoa as a substitute for rice and in salads. You can also sprout the seeds if you prefer to eat a raw diet and use this as a substitute for rice. Sprouting will raise the protein content of the grains

Quinoa is considered a complete protein source due to its impressive amino acid profile. It is also one of the most nutrient dense foods on the planet and contains several anti-inflammatory compounds.

Sprout quinoa rather than cooking it as this will retain the anti-inflammatory compounds which would be destroyed by cooking and it will raise the protein content. This tiny little grain truly deserves its title as a superfood.

PUMPKIN SEED: carotenoids found in pumpkin seeds and the omega-3 fatty acids present in them are being studied for their potential benefits. Men with higher amounts of carotenoids in their diet have less risk for prostate issues. They are a good source of Phytosterols (for lowering cholesterol) and minerals.

SUNFLOWER SEEDS

Sunflower seeds are an excellent source of Vitamin E the body's main antioxidant. A1/3 cup of sunflower seeds will provide you with your daily amount of Vitamin E.

They also contain Phytosterols which help to lower cholesterol and magnesium which helps reduce asthma high blood pressure migraines heart attacks and strokes.

Purchase raw seeds if you can find them and add them to salads or mix up your own raw muesli or granola for breakfast.

FATS AND OILS

Although these fats and oils are healthy and have many benefits you should still exercise a degree of caution when using them. Fats and oils are concentrated sources of calories so using them too liberally will increase your caloric intake significantly while not using them at all means you do not get any of their health benefits.

Do not use oils to cook with. Never use olive oil to cook with. The only fats you should ever consider using to cook with should be those that contain medium chain fatty acids **MCFA** such as those found in coconut oil or clarified organic butter. Yes I did say butter! These oils are very heat stable and will not oxidize as easily as the vegetable oils do when exposed to high temperatures.

Almond avocado walnut and blackcurrant seed oil are all considered "good" fats rich in healthy omega 3 and omega 6 fatty acids. Make sure that your diet contains adequate amounts of these foods so that you do not need to use oils at all.

Use common sense when cooking and only use small amounts. A healthy fat is still a fat!

COCONUT OIL: Coconut oil triglycerides are broken down by the liver into ketones which have proven effective as a treatment for Alzheimer's (the ketones are used as an alternative fuel source by the brain cells which are either insulin resistant or because there is no insulin present and they cannot they absorb glucose for fuel.) Both the heart and brain use ketones as an energy source when necessary.

If you have to have fat in your diet for cooking or frying or in place of butter make sure it is virgin coconut oil. Do not ever use hydrogenated oil or heat-pressed oil under any circumstances.

Coconut oil does raise cholesterol levels. It raises the HDL good cholesterol which helps to remove the LDL bad cholesterol. In other words it is good for you! Studies have shown that populations with diets rich in coconut oil have fewer issues with heart disease.

There is evidence to suggest that coconut oils' benefits may also extend to the treatment of Parkinson's disease epilepsy dementia ALS schizophrenia and autism. On top of all this it is a natural antibiotic that helps to control viruses like HIV and herpes by fighting bacteria so that the immune system can focus on the virus instead. It also helps improve thyroid function.

Coconut oil contains enzymes that assist in its digestion which means that the pancreas does not need to release enzymes. This also helps with the digestion of other foods consumed with coconut oil. 3-6 tablespoons per day is the commonly recommended amount to take if you have a thyroid condition.

Virgin coconut oil is a medium chain fatty acid. It does not need to be broken down by enzymes in the same way that long chain saturated fats are. The liver is damaged by oxidized and rancid oils whether from vegetable or animal origin but this is not the case with coconut oil which is very stable and will not cause any oxidative stress to the liver. .

This will enable the liver to do a better job of converting T4 to T3 which would normally be hampered by the production of other enzymes. Coconut oil is much easier to absorb than seed oils placing less stress on the digestive system and provide energy quicker and requires no insulin to process. Coconut oil acts more like a carbohydrate than a fat but without the sugar high.

The medium chain fats are known as Lauric acid and Myristic acid both of which are found in coconut oil. Medium chain saturated fats are processed by the liver faster than long chain saturated fats. This means that medium chain saturated fats like coconut oil are used for energy while long chain saturated fats are stored rather than used.

Unsaturated fats damage mitochondria by suppressing respiratory enzyme and causing oxidative stress. Unsaturated fats inhibit tissue response to thyroid hormones this suppresses the metabolism by creating hypothyroidism. Unsaturated fats also increase serotonin by allowing tryptophan to enter the brain causing the tired or drowsy feeling.

Seed oils contain plant toxins that target mammalian enzymes. This is the plants defence mechanism to prevent overgrazing. The unsaturated fats block the proteolytic digestive enzyme in the stomach which then prevents the thyroid from creating thyroid hormones. Simply put, unsaturated fats slow down the metabolism. This is not the case with saturated fat from coconuts, which speeds up the metabolism.

Long chain fats are stored in adipose tissue but short chain fats are absorbed into the bloodstream to be used as energy. Medium chain fatty acids easily penetrate cell membranes to fuel the mitochondria.

The thyroid regulates the metabolism. If your thyroid is underactive then you will gain weight. Coconut oil has a long history of use as a fat burning weight loss supplement and by those treating underactive thyroids. It does not cure thyroid issues but acts as a support medium by improving tissue sensitivity to thyroid hormones.

In the 1940s farmers tried fattening livestock up by feeding then cheap coconut oil. It worked in reverse and they got even leaner animals! The health benefits of this unfairly demonized saturated fat have been well known for many decades.

Coconut oil supports thyroid function and since the thyroid controls brain development it also supports healthy brain development. It helps to protect against the anti-thyroid effects of unsaturated fats. There is a fair amount of anecdotal evidence that using coconut oil is beneficial for type 2 diabetics but now there is scientific evidence to back these claims.

In 2009 a study done at Sydney's Garvan Institute of Medical Research [60] has proven that coconut oil will protect against insulin resistance and help prevent weight gain.

BUTYRIC ACID increases the uptake of thyroid hormone into the brain by increasing T3 uptake by the glial cells. It also dilutes and displaces anti-thyroid unsaturated oils. It has blood sugar modulating mitochondria protective and anti-allergy properties. Butyric acid supports the health and healing of cells in both the small and large intestines.

CAPRIC ACID in coconut oil is believed to balance insulin levels and help repair insulin sensitivity.

CAPRYLIC ACID has been used in the treatment of several medical issues such as root canal infection, upper respiratory infection, incontinence, candida albicans infection and wound healing. It also has potential for the treatment of cancer, Alzheimer's and autism. It is also said to improve circulation issues.

LAURIC ACID (dodecanoic acid): a medium chain fatty acid (MCFA) is converted into monolaurin a mono-glyceride compound with **antimicrobial, antiviral anti protozoal** and **antifungal** properties.

Monolaurin targets bacterial infections and lipid-coated (fat-coated) viruses such as measles influenza Herpes Simplex Hepatitis C and HIV and works by destroying the lipid membranes of these organisms and in this way kills them. Lauric acid is an essential fatty acid that is a vital part of the immune system. Monolaurin is a monoglyceride that destroys the cell membranes of lipid (fat) covered viruses such as HIV measles herpes and the flu virus.

Lauric acid is believed to be beneficial in treating skin infections eczema psoriasis and fighting flu viruses and the common cold. It also increases HDL cholesterol. Monolaurin is beneficial to healthy bowel function and digestion. It is anti-allergenic immune boosting and helps to modulate blood sugar.

The body needs Lauric acid to produce monolaurin and the only human source of Lauric acid is breast milk which acts as an artificial immune system for infants. Lauric acid stimulates the immune system and helps to modulate blood sugar levels.

Pure virgin coconut oil contains approximately 50% Lauric acid. Do not freeze coconut oil as this will separate the Lauric acid from the coconut oil.

MYRISTIC ACID (tetradecanoic acid): a medium chain fatty acid is used by the body to stabilize protein including proteins used by the immune system. Myristic acid helps the liver to synthesize cholesterol. Medium chain fatty acids do not circulate in the blood and may increase metabolism.

Populations with a high dietary intake of coconut do not have high cholesterol issues or higher rates of coronary heart disease.

Do not use commercial hydrogenated coconut oil that has been processed into a trans-fat. This is a dangerous fat that has a longer shelf-life for financial reasons with no consideration for your health.

Only use virgin cold-pressed fermented coconut oil. Coconut oil is the only oil recommended for frying if you absolutely must fry at all. Only use small amounts and do not use every day.

MEDIUM CHAIN TRIGLYGERIDES AND WEIGHT LOSS

Medium chain triglycerides (MCTs) or medium chain fatty acids are beneficial in weight loss. MCTs do not need bile to be digested and do not require any energy to be spent on absorption or storage.

MCTs are used as energy almost immediately requiring very little effort from the body to process and have been used as nutritional treatments for many malabsorption illnesses.

Studies have shown that MCTs increase fat oxidation and satiety. MCTs increase energy expenditure and a decrease in the size of fat cells.

They also promote adipose (fat) tissue oxidation. This is when your body uses up stored fat for energy.

A study done in 2007 on free-living diabetics given a daily MCT supplement for 90 days resulted in weight loss and lowered cholesterol levels. The strange contradiction here is that saturated fat sources of medium chain fatty acids like coco nut oil or butterfat (ghee) can lead to weight loss and yet the science does seem to indicate that this is actually true.

This does not imply that more is better. A sensible diet that low in starchy carbohydrates and high in fibre can allow for some MCT rich saturated fats.

Make sure that it is a MCT rich fat like virgin coconut oil. Use a BMR (basal metabolic rate) calculator to work out what your daily caloric needs are to maintain or lose weight and from this you can work out how much saturated fat you are allowed per day.

Drinking Green tea is another way to promote fat oxidation and fat loss.

RED PALM OIL

Red palm oil, or Dende oil, is another plant sourced saturated fat. It has a bright reddish-orange colour and should not be confused with palm kernel oil.

This oil is a relatively new, or at least unknown, fat in the western world. It is used extensively in Africa, Asia and Brazil.

It is rich in alpha-carotene and beta-carotene (vitamin A), lycopene, and tocopherols and tocotrienols (vitamin E). These are all heart friendly phytonutrients.

There is research that proves that daily use of red palm oil will actually decrease cholesterol, rather than raise cholesterol levels despite it being a saturated fat.

Red palm oil may be used in the same way that coconut oil is used. Make sure that you only use cold pressed, virgin red palm oil.

Due to the deforestation of rainforests in Malaysia and Indonesia to plant palm trees, it would be advisable to buy red palm oil ONLY from reputable, sustainable sources.

GRAINS AND PULSES

OATS: Oats and oat bran contain beta-glucan a soluble fibre which has proven ability to lower cholesterol which will help reduce the risk of heart disease. Beta-glucans have been used in treating high cholesterol diabetes asthma H1N1 allergies hepatitis and many more. When eaten it prevents cholesterol from being absorbed from food in the stomach and intestines. When injected, beta-glucan increases chemicals that stimulate the immune system and prevent infection. Oats and oat flour are now considered safe for people with coeliac disease. Oats are a source of Manganese Selenium Magnesium and B vitamins. 1 ½ cups of oats has 3g of beta-glucan soluble fibre. Eating this amount per day can lower cholesterol by 8-23%.

Beta glucan binds with cholesterol and prevents it from getting back to the liver and being reabsorbed. Beta glucan also binds with bile acids and both bile acids and cholesterol are excreted from the body through the feces.

The liver is in charge of making bile from cholesterol so if bile is not around the liver has to go to the blood vessels and get the cholesterol it needs to create more bile. The result is less cholesterol in the blood. Beta-glucan also delays the digestion of carbohydrates. Oats are also a low GI / GL food that will not spike blood glucose levels.

Antioxidants called avenanthramides in oats prevent LDL cholesterol oxidising. They also suppress the production of several types of molecules involved in the attachment of monocytes or immune cells in the bloodstream to the arterial wall which is the first step in the development of atherosclerosis. Vitamin C supplementation increases the strength of avenanthramides health benefits. Oats have a long history of use as an anti-inflammatory. Eat your oats.

LENTILS: lentils are an excellent source of lean protein (30%) and fibre. While dried lentils are an incomplete protein once sprouted they become a complete protein. They are a good source of folate vitamin B1 and iron. Remember to rinse the sprouts regularly to remove phytates.

HERBS AND SPICES

Plain vegetables will have you off the wagon in a matter of weeks from boredom and monotony. Luckily there are options to put a little flavour into the mix with health benefits but without added calories.

All herbs and spices are acceptable however some have more benefit than others. I suggest learning about spice combinations and creating your own blends rather than buying commercial blends that are full of fillers sodium and sugar. Create your own herb mixes for dressings to use on salads and vegetables. Here is a short list of just some of them.

BASIL: contains anti-oxidants like orientin and vicenin high levels of vitamin A, cryptoxanthin, lutein and zeaxanthin. These compounds act as protective scavengers against oxygen-derived free radicals. It also contains essential oils such as eugenol, citronellol, linalool, citral, limonene and terpineol. These compounds are known to have anti-inflammatory and anti-bacterial properties.

BAY LEAF: contains compounds that have antiseptic anti-oxidant digestive and anti-cancer properties. Bay leaves are an excellent source of vitamin A and 100 g. contain 206% of the recommended daily levels of Vitamin A.

BLACK PEPPER: Piperine is a powerful anti-inflammatory and antioxidant and is also believed to increases insulin sensitivity. Piperine stimulates amino acid transporters in the intestinal lining increasing the availability of nutrients from food and supplements. It boosts the availability of curcumin (which is not particularly well absorbed orally) and resveratrol. Piperine in black pepper acts as an antioxidant. Use black pepper with turmeric to boost the absorption of curcumin.

Caution should be used by people taking Digoxin, Lanoxin, Phentoin and Dilantin as it slows down the rate at which the liver removes these medications from the bloodstream.

CAYENNE: Cayenne pepper has been used as a sports supplement for many years to boost the metabolism and improve blood circulation and circulation in general. The active ingredient in chilli is the alkaloid compound **capsaicin** which is a potent anti-inflammatory anti-bacterial anti-carcinogenic analgesic and anti-diabetic agent. Capsaicin stimulates the release of fell-good hormones called endorphins.

Substance P a neuropeptide is also released by capsaicin and has been shown to reverse type 1diabetes in mice. The lab mice who were genetically predisposed to Type 1 diabetes were prevented from developing Type 1 diabetes by removing the TRVP1 neurons which are thought to attract pathogenic T-cells to attacking pancreatic beta cells and so causing type 1diabetes.

Capsaicin was injected into the mice and permanently removed pancreatic sensory neurons which express the Transient Receptor Potential Vanilloid-1 (TRPV1) protein. Insulin resistance and beta cell stress in mice was prevented when TRPV1+ neurons were eliminated.

Reports of its use by Jamaican traditional healers to cure diabetes sparked scientific research into the potential of capsaicin.[61] It was discovered that capsaicin did cause a noticeable drop in blood glucose levels.

 Studies have also shown possible benefit of capsaicin to treat lung cancer prostate cancer and leukaemia. It is used in the treatment of rheumatoid arthritis cardiovascular problems stroke and fibromyalgia.

Capsaicin works by depleting or interfering with Substance P which is a chemical that transmits pain signals to the brain. Capsaicin is available as a medication in pharmacies. It is used by athletes and people suffering from various inflammatory illnesses. Or you could just eat chillies!

Capsaicin has also been reported to lower LDL (bad) cholesterol and blocks the gene that causes arteries to contract causing the muscles to relax and better blood flow to the heart.

Be careful of eating too much however as it can damage the stomach lining. It is available in capsule form as a supplement. A definite must for diabetics!

CARDAMOM: Cardamom has a high anti-oxidant count that helps to restore glutathione levels. Glutathione protects cells against toxins.

CINNAMON: Research has shown that cinnamon has a modest effect in lowering blood glucose levels triglycerides and total cholesterol in type 2 diabetics. Taking cinnamon daily has been shown to reduce cholesterol levels by 18% and blood glucose levels by 24% when 1-6g are consumed daily.

It comes in capsule so you can take it with every meal if you do not like the taste of straight cinnamon. Use caution if you are taking medication or supplements that may lower blood glucose levels as you risk having a hypo if you use too much cinnamon.

FENNEL: Fennel is high in potassium which is important for a reducing salt levels in the body and maintaining a healthy blood pressure. Fennel seeds have many essential oil compounds such as anethole, limonene, anisic aldehyde, pinene, myrcene, fenchone, chavicol and cineole which are known to have antioxidant digestive carminative and anti-flatulent properties.

GARLIC: is believed to boost immunity reduce cholesterol reduce high blood pressure lower blood sugar levels and prevent atherosclerosis. Studies have shown that eating one fresh clove per day can lower your cholesterol by 9% and aged garlic supplements can lower blood pressure by 5.5 %. Allicin in garlic is believed to be the active ingredient responsible for the beneficial health claims.

GINGER: contains essential oils such as gingerol, zingerone, shogaol, farnesene, cineol and citral. Gingerol helps improve intestinal motility and has anti-inflammatory analgesic nerve soothing anti-pyretic as well as anti-bacterial properties. Studies have shown that it may reduce nausea induced by motion sickness or pregnancy and may help relieve migraine headaches. Zingerone which gives ginger its pungent characteristic has been found to be effective against E.coli induced diarrhea especially in children. Use ginger regularly in food juices or as a tea for a healthy digestive system.

THYME: Contains thymol, one of the more important essential oils, which has been found to have antiseptic and anti-fungal characteristics. Thyme also contains many flavonoid Phenolic antioxidants like zeaxanthin, lutein, pigenin, naringenin, luteolin and thymonin giving thyme one of the highest antioxidant levels among herbs.

TURMERIC: Contains Curcumin has an anti-viral anti-fungal anti-bacterial anti-oxidant anti-inflammatory and anti-carcinogenic property. It is well researched in regards to treating several types of cancer such as leukaemia and cancers of the prostate breast and colon. It blocks specific pathways needed for the development of cancers causing cancer cells to "commit suicide".

It promotes wound healing through its antioxidant and anti-inflammatory properties. It appears to be very helpful in the treatment of inflammation emphysema diseases of the cardiovascular system congestive heart failure and gastro-intestinal issues. According to biologists at Tufts University curcumin reduces body weight and cholesterol in overweight animals by shrinking fat cells.

Researchers at UCLA found that it helps prevent tiny blockages in the brain that may cause Alzheimer's; it also increases the expression of enzymes that manufacture gamma-aminobutyric acid (GABA) thereby protecting neurons from oxidative stress.

Studies have shown that curcumin switches on a gene that produces antioxidant proteins. Bilirubin protects the brain against oxidative damage. Curcumin crosses the blood-brain barrier and also induces the expression of a gene called hemeoxygenase-1 (HO-1) produced in the hippocampus.

It is thought that curcumin helps clear out Amyloid Plaque fragments from the brain cells of Alzheimer's patients. The ingredient in curcumin that does this is called bisdemethoxycurcumin and is believed to boost the immune system of Alzheimer's patients.

Black pepper is a symbiotic spice to use with turmeric as it increases the bioavailability of the curcumin in turmeric.

COCAO [62] [63] [64]

Research has shown that chocolate specifically cacao or cocoa has the ability to lower blood pressure and significantly increase insulin sensitivity. Cocoa has heart-friendly flavonoids in particular epicatechin which has been shown to improve circulation and have a beneficial effect on cardiovascular health.

It is loaded with anti-oxidants and polyphenols. In fact cacao has more anti-oxidants per gram than red wine green tea blueberries or goji berries.

It also contains Gallic acid which is anti-viral anti-fungal and anti-oxidant and has shown cytotoxic activity towards cancer cells. It also has Oleic acid the same heart-healthy monounsaturated fat found in olive oil. This makes it useful in lowering LDL cholesterol.

Cocoa is an excellent source of manganese potassium calcium zinc and iron. It also contains beta-carotene, lysine, leucine, lipase, dopamine and anandamide.

Sugar-free is the rational choice and always get the darkest percentage you can around 70-85% the darker the better. There is a debate over the spelling of cocoa but the uneasy consensus is that cocoa is the anglicised spelling and that cacao is the original spelling. There is no such thing as raw cocoa since all cocoa must undergo a heating process to extract cocoa butter which is solid at room temperature.

SALT

Sodium chloride or table salt is made up of 40% sodium and 60% chloride. The heated debate on this topic continues. Yes we need it or no we don't!

The fact is that we cannot live without salt. Blood sweat and tears! It is critical in maintaining the water content in the blood balancing acids and bases and electrical impulses in muscle nerves. The heart liver kidneys adrenal glands and digestive system all need it to some degree.

Too much salt however raises your blood pressure and constricts the arteries. Your heart now has to work twice as hard to pump blood through strangled arteries which is bad news if you have plaque coating the inside of your arteries.

Sodium induced high blood pressure is your body's way of trying to eliminate excess salt. The extra pressure on your arteries if left untreated can lead to heart attacks and strokes.

Sodium also dehydrates blood cells and blood vessels and organs. Lower back ache is often a symptom of the kidneys struggling to cope with too much salt. Too little salt however and you can look forward to diarrhoea nausea vomiting fatigue and lethargy loss of appetite restlessness spasms cramps and irritability.

A 2011 study by Harvard Medical School[65] suggests that too little salt can increase the risks of insulin resistance in only 7 days of commencing a low sodium diet. A similar study by Harvard in 2010 suggests that a low sodium diet may also increase the risks of a cardiac event and death.

An Australian study[66] has shown that type 2 diabetics had higher death rates from cardiovascular events when on low sodium diets.

Another recent study[67] has shown that low sodium diets increase blood cholesterol (2.5%) and triglyceride (7%) levels.

So how much salt do you need per day?

Answer: The opinion on this varies from country to country but the average seems to be a standard teaspoon (2000-2300mg). Many would argue that half this would be fine but that is a matter for discussion with your doctor. The bare minimum is 500mg (1/4 tsp.) for the proper functioning of the body. In Japan the daily average consumption is 6-8 teaspoons of salt in America it is 4-5 teaspoons. That is a lot more than 1 teaspoon!

Natural salts like pink salt and other natural salts are the preferred choices because of their high content of dissolve minerals. Another good choice is Solo salt a reduced sodium (60% less) salt with potassium and magnesium. Other low sodium options are lo-salt and resalt.

These low sodium salts can potentially cause Hyperkalaemia (high blood levels of potassium) in people taking certain drugs or with kidney or heart problems. Diabetics are cautioned not to use them in certain instances so if you are uncertain you need to consult your doctor before using or simply do without.

The argument still rages for and against the use of salt. I feel better when I use salt, but then **I am in control** of how much salt I am using since I no longer eat processed or convenience foods.

 The decision on how much salt you need is between you and your doctor. Choose a good quality natural pink salt and stay away from convenience foods and processed foods that contain processed salts.

You need to be responsible for how much salt is added to your food, not a faceless food manufacturer.

SPROUTED GRAIN FLOUR

Learn to make sprouted grain flour. Grains are an important part of our diets and have been for thousands of years. Bleached, refined, processed flours are a recent addition to our diets and are responsible for a wide selection of health complications. Sprouted grain flour is up to 20 times more nutritious than un-sprouted flour. Sprouting also destroys phytates

Sprouting activates plant enzymes and creates more vita-mins minerals amino acids and protein content within the grain. It also drops the GI of the grain considerably. The starch is broken down into monosaccharide which gets used for growth. Sprouting makes the flour more digestible because your system no longer needs to convert or process the starches.

AT some point you may want to satisfy your carbohydrate cravings. The safest way to do this is with sprouted grain flour. It will not be anything like store bought flour but it will be much healthier

There are several grains to use for sprouted grain flour either individually or in combinations of your choice. Wheat, Spelt, Kamut, Rye, Barley, Oat, Buckwheat ,Millet, etc.

CAUTION:
Wheat will ALWAYS contain **Gluten**. It is the protein component of wheat so if you have trouble with gluten you may want to avoid wheat in favour of the other gluten free grains.

There are reports that people with IBS and coeliacs have found sprouted grains tolerable but this will vary from one person to another. Please also note that sprouted grain flour is *part* of a healthy diet and not *most* of the diet. Use sparingly!

Method for sprouted grain flour

You will need organic whole grains. The choice is yours if you want wheat rye spelt or even a mixture of several different grains.

Soak organic grains in water overnight. Drain. Rinse and drain twice daily for 4 days or until the grains start to grow "tails". Dry in food dehydrator or low fan oven (with door slightly open) overnight or till dry. Grind in flour mill spice mill or coffee grinder.

That was difficult!

Use moisture absorbers when storing the flour and make smaller batches as needed rather than larger batches occasionally. Use the same as for regular flour. Do not expect anything made from sprouted grain to be indistinguishable from regular flour! It will be different enough to notice but similar enough to satisfy cravings.

Products made from sprouted grain keep better in the fridge or freezer.

FERMENTED AND LIVE CULTURE FOODS

Fermented soy products like Miso Natto and Tempeh all support healthy bacteria. There are also fermented vegetables like Sauerkraut and Kimchi to consider.

You may even want to consider making your own rejuvelac drink from fermented grain spouts. These foods all need to be considered as part of a healthy diet. They provide beneficial bacteria for the digestive system which assist in the digestion of foods and the assimilation of nutrients in those foods.

The probiotic bacteria will assist in the digestion of food thus enabling better absorption of nutrients from the food. It will also help repopulate the intestinal flora killed off by eating too much food containing preservatives and chemicals.

Make sure that the fermented food contains live cultures and is not pasteurized since this process kills off the beneficial cultures. There is no benefit to be had from eating dead bacteria. You may want to learn how to make your own live cultured foods, whatever your tastes dictate.

CHEATING

You are going to cheat! I know I did so why should you be any different. If we are going to fall off the wagon occasionally then we should at least have the option of the healthiest possible "bad" choice.

We are social beings and as such we will attend social gatherings where we will not have healthy options. Be smart about your choices and do not stress too much about having a cheat day every once in a while.

Sometime you do not get the option for a "healthy" cheat and then you need to use your own judgement. How much do you enjoy being diabetic? Does the situation call for you to put your life in jeopardy?

The word I like to use is **occasionally** as in *occasion*-ally. Tuesday night on the couch in front of the television with tableful of junk is not an occasion! Weddings, graduations and grandma's 120th birthday are all occasions.

That being said it is acceptable to pig out or gorge once in a while. It seems that having a binge after a week of strict dieting may actually be good for you and that it actually has a beneficial effect on the thyroid.

Timothy Ferriss in his book "The 4 Hour Body" says that a scheduled once a week pig-out day has the effect of balancing the thyroid. This is done once a week after following a strict slow carb low calorie and high fibre diet for six days out of seven.

The risks of this procedure (cheat day binge eating) are as yet unknown for type 2 diabetics. It was never intended to be used by people with a metabolic syndrome so any attempts at doing it are done so at your own risk. If you do attempt it, make certain that you choose healthier, unprocessed cheat foods.

It is possible to minimise the blood glucose spikes caused by binge eating by drinking a small glass of naringen rich grapefruit juice and then doing a few minutes of squats within an hour of bingeing.

Naringen mimics the action of insulin by opening receptors in the muscle cells to allow blood glucose in to fuel the working muscles. What is unknown is whether this will be the case in someone like a type 2 diabetic who is insulin resistant.

THE FINAL WORD

Type 2 diabetes is a chain reaction of metabolic processes that are brought about by poor diet and lack of exercise but it can be reversed. Change the way you eat what you eat and become more physically active and you WILL reverse the effects of type 2 diabetes. Whether or not you remain diabetes free depends entirely on you.

Bariatric surgery, raw vegan diets, vegetarian diets, calorie restricted and low GI/GL diets have all proven effective in reversing diabetes. It is possible and it can be done. The research is out there find it if you still have any doubts.

Diabetes is an incredibly complex disease and has been studied for hundreds, possibly thousands, of years but we are only now scratching the surface of its complexity and yet we still cannot see the forest for the trees.

The cure however is less complex than the disease. We are simply not looking in the right places. The stuff that we call food today is behind the all the trouble. The old saying goes: "you are what you eat". If you eat junk then junk becomes a part of you. It is that simple.

The food we eat is causing us to be unwell. We eat nutrient poor processed foods loaded with trans-fats, synthetic chemicals and sugars. Where are the enzymes, phytochemicals and fibres needed for toxin removal and cell repair?

We eat foods that are stripped down and concentrated with all the naturally occurring safety mechanisms removed. We focus on a narrow selection of foods that cause nutrient deficiencies yet still make us fat. We eat food that is "enriched" with cheap vitamins and minerals because the naturally occurring vitamins have been removed during processing.

We eat foods that we have been assured are healthy for us in large amounts (because they're healthy obviously) only to be told decades later that they are not.

Convenience food is deadly food!

Changing the way we do things is going to be a difficult but life changing process but it is a process that must be done if we are to have a life at all.

The medical profession has told us that diabetes is incurable. It is now telling us that it may be reversible. The facts are too many and too contradictory to know who is telling the truth and who is telling a lie. Science can be used to explain any viewpoint either for or against.

You get to choose what you eat and how you will feel. This is a universe of free will and your choices are yours to make. I made the wrong ones and paid a heavy price. I am now slowly getting back to a condition I only knew when I was a kid before decades of toxic build-up eventually took its toll.

I have used the medical tests done on me to prove the facts that a mostly raw food diet has helped me cure my diabetes. The choices I make post-diabetes are much more considered and educated now.

I wish you the best of luck and the strength in whichever approach you take in reversing your diabetes. It will be difficult but it can be done. The choices you make are yours to make good or bad.

Good health

Jonathan Prins

RAW FOOD
RECIPES

The art of medicine consists of amusing the patient while nature cures the disease

- Voltaire

BREAKFAST
RAW BERRY BIRCHER MUESLI

1 cup oats
1 cup water / oatmilk / almond milk
1tsp cinnamon
2tbsp ground flaxseed
1/2 cup blueberries fresh or defrosted
1 scoop vegetarian protein powder optional

Makes 2-3 servings

Soak oats cinnamon and flaxseed with liquid in a container the night before in the fridge. Add the berries and stir to mix. The mix can also be thinned with water and blended into a breakfast smoothie.

GRANOLA OAT CRUNCH

½ cup uncooked rolled oats
1/3 cup almonds chopped
1/3 cup pumpkin seeds
¼ cup sunflower seeds
¼ cup raw walnuts chopped
¼ cup coconut flakes
1/3 cup pumpkin seeds
1tsp cinnamon
¼ cup chia seeds or ground flaxseed
1 scoop vegetarian protein powder optional

Mix all the ingredients together and store in an airtight container. Serve with oat or almond milk and a few blueberries.

OAT SMOOTHIE

½ cup oats soaked overnight   in 1 ½ cups water
¼ cup sunflower seeds
¼ cup pumpkin seeds
1 tsp. cinnamon
1tbls ground flaxseed
1 scoop vegetarian protein powder optional

Blend in blender adding extra water if needed and drink. Add a few blueberries for variation.

BUCKWHEAT GROATS CEREAL

Sprout 2cups of buckwheat making sure you rinse them regularly at least twice a day. They should be ready in 1-2 days when their "tails" have just appeared. They can be eaten raw or dehydrated.
Dehydrate the groats in the oven on the lowest setting and store them in an airtight container. Or use a dehydrator if you have one. Store the raw groats in the fridge and use within 2-3 days.

 Eat the groats raw or dehydrated with oat or almond milk as a cereal with sunflower seeds pumpkin seeds fresh or frozen berries and chopped nuts adding a sprinkle of cinnamon for flavour.

SALADS

RUSSIAN RED SLAW

2 cups red cabbage grated
1 ½ cups beetroot grated
1 red onion finely chopped
1 Tbls. Flaxseed oil
3 Tbls. Apple cider vinegar
2tsp. caraway seeds optional

Mix together and store in refrigerator will keep for 4-5 days refrigerated.

SAMBAL

1 red onion chopped
1 tomato chopped
1/3 cucumber chopped
1 carrot grated
1 capsicum (bell pepper) chopped
½ bunch cilantro (coriander leaf) chopped
1 tsp. cumin seeds
black pepper to taste
fresh lime juice

When Mix all ingredients together and serve or store in the refrigerator.

SUCCOTASH

1cup raw corn fresh or defrosted
1 red onion chopped
1-2 carrots grated
1-2 celery stalks chopped
1/3 cup sundried tomato soaked drained and chopped
3 Tbls. Apple cider vinegar
1 tsp. oregano herb
black pepper to taste

Mix together and serve or store in the refrigerator.

LENTIL AND QUINOA SALAD

1 cup lentils sprouted
1 cup quinoa sprouted
1 cup carrot grated
½ cup chopped fresh parsley
½ cup red onion chopped
½ cup raw beetroot grated
1 Tbls. Flaxseed oil
3Tbls. Apple cider vinegar

Mix together and serve or store in the refrigerator.

LENTIL TABBOULEH

1 cup quinoa sprouted
1 cup lentils sprouted
½ cup cucumber diced
½ cup tomato diced
½ cup olives chopped
1handful flatleaf parsley chopped
1handful mint leaf chopped
1lemon juiced
1-2 Tbls. cider vinegar optional

Mix all together and serve or store in refrigerator.

THAI YAM PAK SALAD

1 cup carrot shredded
1 cup cabbage finely sliced
1 cup green beans finely sliced
1 red onion thin sliced
½ cup sprouts
2-3 spring onions finely sliced
1 handful mint leaf chopped
1 handful coriander leaf (cilantro) chopped
1 handful basil leaf chopped
DRESSING
1Tbls. fish sauce
2 limes juiced
1tsp. crushed dry chilli or raw sliced chilli

Mix the dressing together and toss through the salad.

CONNIE'S CARROT AND COCONUT SALAD

3 cups grated carrot
1cup fresh coconut grated
1/3 cup raisins
1/3 Walnut pieces

Mix all together. This salad does not need any dressing. Do not be too generous with the raisins as they do contain fructose you may leave them out if you wish.

THAI CARROT SALAD

3 Carrots grated
1/3 cup cashew nuts
1 lime juiced
2 cloves garlic crushed
chilli fresh or dry as much as you can handle in a dish
2 Tbls. fish sauce (optional, omit if you are a vegan)

This salad can be made with green pawpaw / papaya or daikon / mooli /Japanese radish instead if you choose. Blend the lime, chilli, garlic and fish sauce and dress the carrots and cashew nuts with it. Garnish with mint and / or coriander leaf (cilantro).

CAESAR SALAD

1 individual salad portion cos (romaine) lettuce hearts
1/3 cup raw walnuts
black pepper to taste
Woody's Caesar dressing to taste.
Vegan parmesan cheese to taste

Dress the salad with Caesar dressing (on page 278) and serve.

SPINACH AND WALNUT SALAD

Individual portion of baby spinach leaves or Mesclun leaves
1/3 cup walnuts
¼ red onion sliced finely
1 celery stalk sliced finely
1 Tsp. extra virgin olive oil
3 Tbls. Apple cider vinegar

Dress the salad and serve. You can use a simple olive oil dressing or you can use the raw vegan Caesar dressing.

CHEF SALAD

Mixed salad greens, as much as you need for your meal, mixed tomatoes, capsicums, red onion, cucumber, grated carrot, sprouts, sliced green beans, olives, vegan cheese and any other vegetables of your choice.

Dress with apple cider vinegar or lemon juice and a tsp. of virgin olive oil.

A chef salad is essentially a clear-out of the fridge. There are no rules in creating a chef salad and you can be as creative as you want with whatever you find in the fridge (so long as it is raw and vegan).

Be creative!

WOODY'S CAESAR DRESSING

A

5 tablespoons raw tahini

1/4 cup pine nuts

1-2 clove garlic crushed

2 green onions or 1/4 cup sweet red onion

1 lemon juiced

3 tablespoons apple cider vinegar

3softdatespitted and soaked

3tablespoons nutritional yeast

1-2 teaspoon black pepper or to taste

B

1-2 teaspoons sea salt or to taste

2 tablespoons good olive oil (optional)

fresh water 2 tablespoons at a time as necessary to blend.

Blend ingredients listed under **A** together in a blender adding oil and fresh water 2 tablespoons at a time as necessary to blend until very smooth.

Makes 500ml (1 pint) of thick dressing. Thin out if needed.

SPICED VINEGAR

1 litre apple cider vinegar
1-2 bay leaves
1 Tbls. black peppercorns
1 Tbls. allspice/pimento berries
½ Tbls. cloves
1-3 cloves garlic whole or sliced

Place all together in a glass bottle and store in warm dark place for a week for flavour to develop. This can be used to add flavour to salads.

HERB VINEGAR

1 litre apple cider vinegar
1 Tbls. dried thyme
1 Tbls. dried oregano
1 Tbls. black peppercorns
1-2 garlic cloves whole or sliced

Store in the fridge in a glass bottle and allow to develope for a week. Use any combination of herbs you prefer. These are just examples to show how easy it is to add flavour without using oil or commercially prepared dressings.

PLAIN TOMATO SAUCE

1 ½ cups sundried tomatoes soaked
1-2 clove garlic crushed
1tsp. oregano herb
1tsp. basil herb
1Tbls. apple cider vinegar
salt & pepper to taste

Puree in a blender adding water as needed to thin out.
Serve or store in the refrigerator. Serve with crudités or
raw pasta.

CREAMY TOMATO SAUCE

1 cup plain tomato sauce
1 cup soaked cashew nuts drained

Puree together in a blender or processor adding water carefully to desired consistency. Serve with crudités or raw
pasta.

TOMATO TAPENADE

1 cup sundried tomatoes soaked and drained
1 clove garlic crushed
1/3 cup black olives pitted
½ cup of raw cashew nuts unsoaked
¼ tsp. each of basil and oregano herbs

Process in a blender or food processor and serve with crudités or raw zucchini pasta.

MOROCCAN TOMATO DIP

11/2 cups sundried tomatoes soaked
1tsp cinnamon
1tsp Cumin
1tsp coriander
1tsp paprika
½ tsp. turmeric
1-2 cloves garlic crushed
¼ cup parsley chopped
Salt & pepper to taste

Puree together in a blender and serve or store in the refrigerator. Serve with crudités or raw pasta. This can also be thinned out with water and used as a salad dressing.

SMOKEY TOMATO DIP

1 ½ cup sundried tomatoes soaked
1-2 clove garlic crushed
1tsp. smoked paprika
1tsp. oregano herb
1 tsp. cumin powder
1 tsp. coriander powder
black pepper to taste
1Tbls. apple cider vinegar

Puree in a blender and serve or store in the refrigerator. Serve with crudités or raw pasta.

RAW HUMMUS

1 ½ cups sprouted chickpeas rinsed drained and skinned
1-2 clove garlic crushed
1tsp. cumin powder
1tsp.coriander powder
¼ tsp. turmeric powder
¼ cup raw tahini (or make sesame paste)
1lemon juiced
salt & black pepper to taste
garnish with paprika

OPTIONAL

2 cups fresh spinach leaves
1cup fresh basil leaves
1/3 cup sundried tomatoes soaked and drained
2 Tbls. smoked paprika
Add these singly or in combination to the other ingredients
when processing for a variation of flavour.

To sprout chickpeas soak them overnight and then rinse
and drain 2-3 times per day for 3 days. You need to do this
or they will taste bitter. Sprout them too long and they will
taste earthy and "sprouty". Puree all together in a blender
adding water as needed to thin out. Serve or store in the refrigerator

ZUCCHINI DIP

2 large zucchini chopped
½ cup lemon juice
1 tsp. salt
1 ½ tsp. cumin powder
1tsp. coriander powder
1/2 cup raw tahini
½ avocado
1Tbls. White Miso

Puree in a blender adding water if needed. Serve or store in refrigerator. Serve with carrot sticks, celery sticks, etc.

GUACAMOLE

2 avocados scooped
1 spring onion chopped
1handful coriander leaf (cilantro) chopped
1lime juiced
1chilli pepper, chopped

Mix or process all the ingredients together adding seasoning to taste. Eat immediately as it does oxidize easily if stored. Serve on vegetable sticks or dehydrated vegetable crisps

VEGAN CEESES

VEGAN CREAM CHEESE

2 cups raw cashews soaked overnight and drained
1lemon juiced
2Tbls. apple cider vinegar
3probiotic capsules (contents only)
2 Tbls. nutritional yeast
½ tsp. salt
1cup filtered water

Puree everything together in a blender until smooth. Add water in a stream until the desired consistency is achieved adding more water if needed but be careful not to make the mixture runny. Pour into a steel thermos flask or sealable container and allow to stand for a day to develope. Transfer to a storage container and refrigerate.

This cheese may also be strained through cheesecloth and pressed to make a soft cheese.

VEGAN CHEESE

2 cups raw nuts soaked (use macadamia cashew or skinned almonds).
2 Tbls. nutritional yeast
3capsules probiotics (contents only)
1lemon juiced
½ tsp. salt

Optional flavourings:
(1) 1tsp. smoked paprika ¼ tsp. turmeric powder
(2) 1tsp. cracked pepper 1tsp. oregano 1 tsp. basil

Puree all together in a blender with just enough water to ensure smooth blending. Pour into a cheesecloth (or dish-towel) –lined bowl. Squeeze to drain. Add any flavouring mixes at this point and mix well. Place in a colander with a weight on top. Allow to drain for 24 hours at room temperature. Place into a container that you want your cheese to be shaped and allow to set in the refrigerator. It keeps for about a week.

The liquid that is drained off may be drunk as a vegan yoghurt style drink as it contains probiotic culture. Consider adding it to nut or oatmilk as a vegan yoghurt smoothie drink.

VEGAN PARMESAN

1 cup raw nuts (skinless almonds, pine nuts or cashews)
3 Tbls. Nutritional yeast
1tsp. salt
½ tsp. white pepper

Grind all ingredients together in a spice mill or blender.
Spread out on a sheet and dehydrate in the oven on the
lowest temperature (below 40°C / 104°F) or use a dehydrator if you have one. Store in an airtight container.

You can use this on raw pasta or sprinkle it on salads sliced
tomato etc.

SOUPS AND MEALS

WOODY'S MISO SOUP

Serves 2-4
1 medium avocado
2 Roma tomatoes or 1 regular tomato seeded
2 cups coconut water
1 lemon juiced
2 tablespoons white miso
2 tablespoons red miso (or use 4 Tbls. of either)
miso total or only 3 tablespoons red miso total.)
1 tablespoon minced ginger
1 clove garlic
1/2 cup water or as necessary to thin
3 tablespoons parsley chopped

1/4 cup green onion outer skin removed and finely sliced

4 tsp. hulled hemp seed or sesame seeds

Blend avocado tomato coconut water lemon juice miso garlic and ginger until smooth. Add 1/2 cup or more fresh water as necessary to thin the soup to desired consistency. Add chopped parsley and blend for several pulses until mixed in. Sprinkle with chopped green onion and hemp seeds or sesame.

Serve room temperature or gently warmed. This soup also makes a great dipping sauce.

CONNIE'S CURRIED CARROT SOUP

1 avocado

1 tomato

3 celery stalks

1 small red onion

½ bunch of parsley

½ inch piece of ginger

1 tsp. turmeric powder or fresh grated turmeric root

1 tsp. curry powder1

1 lemon juiced

1½ cups carrot juice or coconut water or filtered water

Blend all together in a blender and serve or store in the refrigerator.

GAZPACHO

1 cucumber chopped
4 ripe tomatoes
½ capsicum pepper
2 cloves garlic
3 celery stalks chopped
1 Tbls lemon juice
1/2 red onion chopped
3 Tbls. balsamic or apple cider vinegar
salt and pepper to taste
1 tsp. chopped fresh parsley
tsp. chopped fresh basil
¼ tsp. cayenne pepper or a dash of hot sauce optional

Blend all together in a blender adding water as needed to thin out if so desired. This will keep in the fridge for a few days. This may be eaten as a cold soup or drunk as a Virgin Mary style smoothie

If you intend eating it as a cold soup you can add soaked drained sundried tomatoes to the blender. This will give a thicker texture and stronger flavour. Season with regular or smoked paprika for a little extra flavour.

RAW PASTA

2-3 medium sized straight zucchini
½ cup tomato sauce/dip
black pepper to taste
nutritional yeast to taste
garnish with vegan parmesan and chopped parsley

Using a vegetable peeler slice the zucchini lengthways. If you have a mandolin or a spiral slicer you can make raw spaghetti. Dress the "pasta" with the sauce and then season with salt black pepper and vegan parmesan or nutritional yeast. Eat and enjoy.

SIDE NOTE: you can also dress this "pasta with the Caesar dressing or the Smokey tomato dip for variation.

RAW GREEN BEAN CURRY

2 cups green beans trimmed and sliced
1 cup tomato chopped
1tsp. turmeric ½
tsp. fresh black pepper
1tsp. fresh ginger grated
1tsp. cumin seeds
½ cup of any of the tomato sauces
salt black pepper and cayenne pepper to taste

Mix all together adding green beans and chopped tomatoes last.

HOT DRINKS

ROOIBOS TEA

This herbal tea from South Africa is high in anti-oxidants such as aspalathin and nothofagin. It has no caffeine and very low tannin levels compared to regular tea.

 Rooibos also contains phenolic compounds including flavanols flavones flavanones and dihydrochalcones. It has no oxalic acid making it a safe choice for people with kidney stones. It is rich in minerals like iron calcium potassium copper fluoride manganese zinc and magnesium.

Brew tea and drink hot with a slice of lemon or refrigerate and drink as iced tea with lemon. It is also available as a spiced chai. Sweeten with stevia if you must but it is not a bitter tea at all.

This is a very versatile tea and even has a sweetish taste so you will not need any sweetener at all. It can be drunk hot or turned into iced tea and garnished with lemon.

DECAFFEINATED COFEE

Decaffeinated coffee contains caffeic acid (antioxidant anti-carcinogenic phenol) chlorogenic acid (antioxidant antifungal antiviral and antibacterial that reportedly reduces glucose production by the liver) and ferulic acid (an anti-inflammatory antioxidant that lowers blood glucose blood cholesterol and triglyceride levels). Ferulic acid has been shown to reduce brain inflammation thereby reducing the risks of both Parkinson's and Alzheimer's diseases.

Decaf also contains magnesium and chromium which help diabetics regulate insulin and blood sugar.

In the past there were concerns over the use of chemicals used to extract caffeine from the beans. Today either the "swiss water" method or CO2 gas are used to decaffeinate coffee.

As with regular coffee decaf should not be consumed in excessive amounts either as it does create an acidic environment in the body due to its high acid content. It can over-stimulate the secretion of gastric acids causing reflux.

There is research to suggest that due to decaf being made from a different variety of coffee bean (robusta) which contains a higher level of diterpenes decaffeinated coffee may actually increase LDL (bad) cholesterol levels. Diterpenes (specifically cafestol and Kahweol) are believed to stimulate the production of fatty acids and raise cholesterol levels.

Using paper filters to make coffee instead of a plunger or other style of coffee machine is thought to prevent the diterpenes oils from going into the coffee. If no filter is used then all of the diterpenes are ingested.

The point I am trying to make here is that moderation is to be exercised and that anything, even apparently healthy, can have serious negative side effects. 1-2 cups per day as a supplement to your 6-9 glasses of water is perfectly safe (if you use a paper filter) even beneficial.

HINT: add a tsp. of cinnamon to your coffee filter just before adding the water for a tasty blood sugar lowering treat. Chill the coffee and add oatmilk for an iced coffee on warm days.

DECAFFEINATED GREEN TEA

Decaffeinated green tea contains polyphenols (antioxidants that protect cells from free-radical damage). You still get all the benefits of drinking green tea but without the negatives of caffeine.

The main polyphenol in green tea is a catechin called **Epigallocatechin-3-gallate (EGCG)** and it helps prevent the death of heart muscle cells. **EGCG** also protects the pancreatic beta cells from the cytotoxic effects of IAPP fibrils. It has also been used as a treatment for diabetes in lab animals.

It is also believed to be of benefit in fighting several types of cancer heart disease gum disease lowering blood pressure and triglycerides protecting brain cells by preventing the formation of free radicals in the brain tissue and preventing the development of atherosclerosis.

Make sure that you only buy tea that has been decaffeinated using the CO2 method and not the ethyl acetate method. If in doubt find out!

The psychological benefits of enjoying a cup of green tea or a cup of coffee do not need to be spoiled by the effects of caffeine anymore. This is not a permit to consume as much as you like since polyphenols will interfere with iron absorption.

It does mean that you can now enjoy a cup of green tea (or two) or a cup of coffee (or two) without feeling guilty anymore!

HINT: Add a slice of lemon to your tea instead of (oat) milk and chill it for iced tea. Add mint leaves for a middle-eastern style tea.

HOT CHOCOLATE

1Tbls.cocoa powder
½ tsp. cinnamon

Add hot water to mix and stevia if you need in to be sweet. Add nut or oat milk if you like it milky. You can also add a spoon of coconut oil for added richness.

Cocoa has health benefits in the form of antioxidants and neurotransmitters but it also contains the stimulant theobromine which has a similar chemical structure to caffeine

Theobromine is a vasodilator (it opens the blood vessels allowing blood to flow freely) and a heart stimulant. It has been used in the treatment of high blood pressure. It is also a diuretic.

Enjoy your cocoa but do not consume more than once per day as it can have similar effects as caffeine.

CAUTION: polyphenols found in coffee green tea and cocoa can inhibit iron absorption so be aware of this if you do drink them regularly.
Have your iron levels checked regularly and supplement accordingly if recommended by your doctor or healthcare advisor.

COLD DRINKS

RYE REJUVELAC

Rejuvelac is a raw fermented drink that will assist with digestion. It is a probiotic fermented drink.

2 cups whole rye grains
filtered water

Soak the rye for 12 hours in cool water. Rinse and drain well.

Sprout the rye rinsing twice daily for 24 hours

Add 6 cups of water to sprouted rye and let it stand uncovered somewhere out of the way for 2 days.

Strain off the water and save it. This is the rejuvelac. The rye grains may be used to make a second batch but not a third. The rye grains may now be composted or fed to the birds.

Store the rejuvelac in the fridge. The taste does grow on you.

COCONUT WATER

Coconut water contains only 70 calories per 310ml / 10.5 FL.OZ. (Approximately 45 calories per cup). It does contain coconut sugar which means that you do need to restrict the amount you consume to only 3 per week at most if you are sweating from exercise.

It is a very good natural electrolyte solution and makes a good substitute for fruit juice or soda if you are struggling to avoid cheating. It contains potassium chloride sodium phosphorous manganese and calcium. It is also full of amino acids vitamins antioxidants and Lauric acid. All in all a much better choice than commercial sports drinks since it is a natural electrolyte.

It contains cytokinins which are plant hormones that slow the aging process in plants and fruit flies. There is a belief that this might also be the case for people. Potassium helps to lower blood pressure and improves heart health.

COCONUT SMOOTHIE

1 drinking coconut juice and pulp

Blend everything together into a smooth consistency and drink as is or over ice. This is a high calorie drink that makes 2 portions so do not drink the entire batch all at once. Save the other half in the fridge for a few days' time.

These are also called Thai coconuts or young coconuts and are widely available. Most supermarkets and greengrocers have them.

They are a good source of electrolytes and some fatty acids and amino acids.

VAMPIRO

1 large beetroot
2 large carrots
½ cucumber
3 celery stalks

Juice and drink immediately. This juice is a liver cleanser and blood purifier. Once or twice a week should be enough any more than that and you risk getting too much iron magnesium copper and phosphorous.

Betalaine is the phytochemical that causes beetroot to be so red. It is also what causes beeturia when you go to the loo afterwards and panic when you see red. Do not worry this is harmless and normal.

Beeturia is more common in people with iron deficiency so you may want to get tested for iron deficiency if you have red urine after eating or drinking beets.

Betaine is a phytochemical found in beetroot. It has been found to lower blood levels of homocysteine. Elevated homocysteine levels are markers for several diseases such as heart disease, kidney disease, Alzheimer's and even schizophrenia. High levels of blood homocysteine are also connected with bone brittleness in elderly people.

Blood pressure can be lowered significantly with a daily glass of beetroot juice. Beetroot is rich in nitrates. Vegetables take nitrates in through their roots. Beetroot is particularly rich in nitrates.

Nitrates are converted into nitric oxide which has vasodilation properties, i.e. it relaxes and opens the blood vessels up. This means that beetroot juice is good for your heart and good for lowering blood pressure.

Research has shown that drinking 250ml of beetroot juice[68] per day can drop blood pressure by up to 10 points, which is better than any medication could do for the same result.

With all these benefits it would seem to be unwise to NOT have a glass of beetroot juice daily.

The secret is to make sure that you drink raw beetroot juice since cooking or processing will destroy many of the phytonutrients in the vegetable or juice.

RAW VEGETABLE JUICES

Raw vegetable juices are a fantastic way to get in massive amounts of phytonutrients, vitamins and minerals in one gulp. Mix and match vegetables to juice as you need. Consult a nutritionist or dietician to get an idea of what your specific nutritional needs might be.

Remember to not overdo it on any one vegetable and to keep things varied to avoid overdosing on anything. Keep it varied in order to get a good avoid toxic overdose of any particular nutrients.

Watch Joe Cross' movie **"Fat, Sick and Nearly Dead"** to get an idea of what vegetable juicing can do for you.

http://www.rebootwithjoe.com/about/fat-sick-and-nearly-dead/

If your doctor clears you to do so, you may want to try a 3-7 day juice fast using only raw vegetable juices. This is a good way to detox and get a solid dose of phytonutrients into your body.

Avoid adding fruit to your juices for the first 30 days so that you minimise your fructose intake.

Raw vegetable juices pack a powerful nutritional punch. Make sure that you get a well-rounded selection of vegetables to juice and do not focus too much on any one particular vegetable.

THE GREEN SMOOTHIE

Green smoothies usually have some form of sweet fruit in them to make them a bit more palatable. This particular smoothie is all about nutrition and does not focus on sweetness.

½ avocado
1 cup chopped, mixed, leafy green vegetables (remember to rotate your leafy green vegetables and not focus on any one particular vegetable)
1 tomato
½ cucumber
½ cup filtered water or juice and flesh of a young coconut
1 scoop vegetarian protein powder optional
juice of 1 lemon

Blend all together in a blender and drink immediately. It makes a quick nutrient-dense meal for breakfast or lunch.

This was not one of my favourite drinks I'll be honest but I did drink them (quickly) because they were an excellent way to get my daily dose of greens down fast.

I had to remind myself that indulging in sweet juices was what got me into trouble and that drinking this was what was going to get me out of trouble. It worked too! At a later stage I began to add whole fruit for nutritional value.

TREATS

I include a section on treats because I have a sweet tooth! I know that many others do too and the urge to satisfy that should be acknowledged and healthy choices provided so that we do not go out and buy unhealthy foods. I did not know of these recipes when I started and fell off the wagon a few times when the sweet cravings took over. Do not make the same mistakes that I did.

Put the effort into making these and save them for when you just cannot stand it anymore. Use willpower to hold out for as long as you can.

Treats should be seen as treats! They are not for every day or whenever you fell like it. Set aside times and places that are your "treat times" and allow yourself to look forward to them and savour the moment when it does arrive. Once or twice per week is fine you can even substitute a piece of whole fruit for a treat since it contains fibre. No fruit juice!

Having a treat occasionally will help with the psychological aspects of cravings and should also prevent the down-regulation of thyroid hormones. Over-consumption however will delay or even stop the reversal process and add fructose which is something we do not want to do.

Some of these treats contain fruits which mean they contain fructose and while that is a bad thing they are completely natural and contain fibre which slows down the absorption rate of fructose.

These recipes were chosen because they contain ingredients that have beneficial health properties but you should still exercise restraint when it comes to fruit and other sweet foods. If you are strong willed you can leave them out completely.

YACON BROWNIES

3/4 cup cacao powder

3 tablespoons ground chia seeds

1 cup almonds soaked skinned and processed

2-3 medjool dates pitted and soaked

3 Tbls. yacon syrup or powder

1 cup shredded coconut

½ teaspoon vanilla or ½ vanilla pod scraped

½ cup Walnuts optional added after blending

mix all the ingredients together in a blender or processor and press into a brownie dish. Cling wrap and allow to set in the fridge overnight.

SWEET VEGAN TARTS

BASE:

1 cup raw almond /macadamia / Brazil nut flour your choice

1cup shredded coconut

2-3 medjool dates pitted and soaked

3 Tbls. extra virgin coconut oil melted

2-3 Tbls. yacon powder optional

2 Tbls. chia seeds

If you are using whole nuts grind them to flour beforehand making sure that you do not turn them into nut butter.
Mix all the other ingredients together making sure that the dates are well mashed and blended. You should have a pliable mixture that is not too smooth. Press into tart trays or a slice pan and refrigerate while you make fillings.

BERRY FILLING

1 cup of berries fresh or defrosted your choice
3 tsp. chia seeds
2Tbls. psyllium husk powder
½ cup Irish moss gel
1apple grated and pureed smooth
1lemon zested and juiced
2 Tbls. melted coconut oil
Mix all the ingredients together in a bowl or blender and pour into tart crusts. Allow   to set in fridge

CHOCOLATE FILLING

1 cup cashew nuts soaked and drained
½ cup cocoa powder
5Tbls melted coconut oil
3 medjool dates pitted and soaked
¾ cup Irish moss gel
3 Tbls. chia seeds
2Tbls. psyllium husk powder
Blend all together in a blender and pour into tart crusts. Allow to set in the refrigerator.

These are just a few examples of raw food cuisine that you can make at home and some of the foods that I ate when reversing my diabetes.

The emphasis should be on raw fresh organic foods wherever possible. I do not have the finances to allow for organic all the time but I try to observe this as much as my finances will allow. If the vegetables I buy are not organic they get washed well to rid them from any pesticide residues.

There are many online resources available to try out and draw inspiration from. Most of us me included struggle to give up cooked foods and meat. The trick is to take small steps and not jump in at the deep end (unless you have the willpower). Add raw foods to your menu in stages until you are eating more raw than cooked.

Reduce meat consumption as much as possible if you cannot go completely vegetarian. I cannot claim to be a vegetarian but consume much less animal protein than I used to.

Avoid starchy and refined carbohydrates (sugar fructose wheat rice etc.) like the plague! Diets high in these foods in conjunction with high dietary intake of trans-fats and poly-unsaturated fats are leading us all down the road to heart disease and diabetes.

Some monounsaturated fats (olive oil) and some medium chain saturated fats (virgin coconut oil) in your diet is acceptable and healthy but be careful not to overindulge. Too much of a good thing can be a bad thing. Try to use fats raw for salad dressings only and not for frying as this can turn them carcinogenic.

Good health and good luck!

Jonathan Prins.

BIBLIOGRAPHY

Barnard, Neal D, M.D.   "Dr Neal Barnard's program for reversing Diabetes" Rodale 2007

Cousens, Gabriel, MD   "There is a Cure for Diabetes" North Atlantic Books 2008
"Rainbow Green Live-Food Cuisine" North Atlantic Books 2003

Ferriss, Timothy   "The 4 hour Body" Vermillion 2011

Gaby, Alan R, M.D.   "The A-Z Guide to Drug-Herb-Vitamin Interactions:" Healthnotes Inc.
"The natural Pharmacy" Healthnotes Inc. 2006

Gross, Paul, Ph.D.   "Superfruits" McGraw- Hill 2010

Holford, Patrick.   "Beat Stress and Fatigue" Piatkus Books 2010
"Optimum Nutrition Made easy" Piatkus Books 2008
"Say No to Diabetes" Piatkus 2011

Massey, Alexandra.   "Superfoods to Boost your mood" Virgin Books Ltd 2006

McCulley, De Wayne.   "Death To Diabetes Version 3.0" Booksurge 2008

Richards, Byron J.   "The leptin Diet: How Fit Is Your Fat?"

Truth in Wellness 2006

Yudkin, John   "Pure White and Deadly" Penguin Books 1988

INDEX

138, 139, 140, 149, 150, 151, 154, 187, 190, 192, 193, 195, 206, 209, 210, 230, 231, 233, 250, 252, 254, 264, 265, 268, 272, 273, 277, 295, 297, 298, 300, 301, 303, 304, 312, 314, 316, 329, 365

Fructosamine, 78

fructose, **21, 27, 34, 35, 40, 41, 43, 62, 79, 81, 89, 90, 93, 94, 95, 96, 100, 109, 120, 126, 138, 139, 140, 148, 153, 190, 200, 208, 209, 233, 237, 251, 260, 265, 267, 268, 272, 277, 297, 340, 365, 368**

fruit, **21, 29, 34, 89, 90, 93, 94, 95, 96, 99, 114, 122, 126, 127, 138, 140, 184, 193, 194, 208, 209, 214, 223, 224, 225, 228, 265, 267, 277, 296, 297, 302, 360, 364, 365, 366**

G

GABA, 59, 286, 321

ghrelin, **96, 151, 152, 155**

GI, **12, 14, 56, 64, 95, 101, 104, 106, 114, 120, 122, 124, 127, 137, 139, 153, 154, 222, 238, 247, 248, 249, 250, 251, 252, 254, 265, 266, 284, 315, 326, 330**

Glucagon, **11, 65, 68, 69**

glucose, **8, 9, 11, 20, 21, 22, 28, 29, 30, 48, 49, 50, 51, 53, 54, 55, 56, 57, 65, 66, 67, 68, 69, 70, 73, 76, 77, 79, 90, 91, 92, 93, 96, 100, 101, 102, 103, 104, 107, 108, 110, 127, 138, 139, 145, 149, 151, 162, 163, 164, 165, 167, 175, 186, 187, 188, 200, 202, 210, 227, 231, 232, 233, 239, 245, 246, 251, 255, 256, 260, 265, 266, 273, 275, 279, 280, 281, 282, 284, 287, 289, 290, 291, 297, 298, 302, 307, 315, 318, 319, 330, 356**

GMO, 271

H

HbA1c, 7, 77, 78, 137, 183, 228, 231, 232, 249, 255, 264, 282

HDL, 49, 82, 83, 84, 94, 112, 113, 119, 294, 299, 301, 307, 311

heart, **5, 27, 41, 47, 48, 49, 58, 59, 60, 66, 69, 73, 74, 78, 83, 84, 94, 96, 100, 107, 108, 109, 110, 111, 112, 113, 114, 118, 119, 132, 138, 140, 143, 145, 162, 164, 166, 167, 169, 173, 174, 179, 186, 200, 227, 233, 239, 256, 266, 275, 280, 282, 283, 285, 286, 288, 292, 294, 297, 299, 303, 305, 307, 312, 314, 318, 321, 322, 323, 325, 357, 358, 360, 368**

high fructose corn syrup (HFCS), **21**

homocysteine, **49, 73, 102, 132, 292**

hyperinsulinemia, **23, 55, 104, 111**

I

IAPP, **8, 9, 289, 357**

IGF-1, 105, 106

inflammation, **10, 21, 22, 30, 56, 57, 58, 59, 60, 61, 62, 67, 85, 96, 102, 104, 131, 140, 142, 143, 144, 146, 161, 163, 173, 174, 178, 239, 268,** 271, **274, 281, 298, 299, 321, 356**

inflammatory response, 24, 56, 271

insulin, **1, 2, 7, 8, 9, 10, 11, 19, 20, 21, 22, 23, 29, 30, 43, 47, 49, 53, 54, 55, 57, 58, 63, 64, 65, 67, 68, 69, 73, 76, 83, 91, 94, 95, 96, 101, 102, 103, 104, 110, 111, 113, 143, 148, 150, 153, 163, 166, 173, 187, 200, 202, 209, 228, 233, 235, 238, 239, 251, 256, 272, 275, 281, 282, 284, 285, 286, 287, 288, 289, 290, 291, 292, 302, 307, 308, 310, 317, 322, 330, 356**

interleukin-6 (IL-6), 162, 173

Islet Amyloid Polypeptide, 8

J

Jim Healthy, **ii, 13, 205**

T

U

V

W

REFERENCES

[1] Reversal of type 2 diabetes: normalisation of beta cell
function in association with decreased pancreas
and liver triacylglycerol,
Diabetologia, DOI 10.1007/s00125-011-2204-7, 2011
E. L. Lim, et al

[2] Type 2 diabetes: remission in just a week,
Diabetologia (2011) 54:2477–2479
DOI 10.1007/s00125-011-2266-6
H. Yki-Järvinen

[3] Reversal of type 2 diabetes: normalization of beta cell function in association
with decreased pancreas and liver triacylglycerol
Diabetologia, Volume 54, Number 10, 2506-2514
R.Taylor , E. L. Lim et al

[4] Activation of the NLRP3 inflammasome by islet amyloid polypeptide provides
a mechanism for enhanced IL-1β in type 2 diabetes
Nature Immunology,Volume:11,Pages:897–904 , 2010
Luke O'Neil, et al

[5] Evidence That Nasal Insulin Induces Immune Tolerance to Insulin in Adults
With Autoimmune Diabetes
Diabetes , April 2011 60:1237-1245; 2011
Spiros Fourlanos, et al

[6] JNK1 in Hematopoietically Derived Cells Contributes to Diet-Induced In-
flammation and Insulin Resistance without Affecting Obesity p386
Cell Metabolism, 7 November, 2007 Volume 6, Issue 5
Giovanni Solinas, et al

[7] Gamma-aminobutyric acid inhibits T cell autoimmunity and the development
of inflammatory responses in a mouse type 1 diabetes model.
J Immunol. 173(8):5298-304. 2004
Tian J, et al

[8] Effect of Dopamine Receptor DRD2 and ANKK1 Polymorphisms on Dietary
Compliance, Blood Pressure, and BMI in Type 2 Diabetic Patients
Shahad Abdulnour
University of Toronto, 2010

9 Unexpected evidence for active brown adipose tissue in adult humans
   AJP - Endo August 2007 vol. 293 no. 2 E444-E452
   Jan Nedergaard

10 Brown adipose tissue: function and physiological significance.
   Physiol Rev. 2004.
   Cannon B, Nedergaard J.

11 Cannabinoid receptor 1 (CB1) antagonism enhances glucose utilisation and
   activates brown adipose tissue in diet-induced obese mice
   Diabetologia Volume 54, Number 12, 3121-3131,
   Sylvana Obici, et al.

12 The role of exercise and PGC1α in inflammation and chronic disease
   Nature 454, 463-469
   Christoph Handschin1 & Bruce M. Spiegelman

13 Increased consumption of refined carbohydrates and the epidemic of type 2
   diabetes in the United States: an ecologic assessment
   Am J Clin Nutr 2004 79: 774-779
   Lee S Gross,et al

14 How safe is fructose for persons with or without diabetes?
   American Journal of Clinical Nutrition, Vol. 88, No. 5, 1189-1190, November
    2008
   Laura Gabriela Sánchez-Lozada, et al

15 Sugar: The Bitter Truth
   Professor Robert H. Lustig
   http://www.youtube.com/watch?v=dBnniua6-oM

16 Sugar: The Bitter Truth (the SHORT version)
   Sean Croxton
   http://www.youtube.com/watch?v=tdMjKEncojQ
   www.Undergroundwellness.com

17 Hyperuricemia in Childhood Primary Hypertension
   Hypertension. 2003; 42: 247-252
   Daniel I. Feig, Richard J. Johnson

18 Basic Science for Clinicians, Advanced Glycation End Products, Sparking the
   Development of Diabetic Vascular Injury
   Circulation. 2006; 114: 597-605 doi: 10.1161/ CIRCULAIOHA.106.621854
    Mark A. Creager, et al.

[19] Coffee acutely modifies gastrointestinal hormone secretion and glucose tolerance in humans: glycemic effects of chlorogenic acid and caffeine
Am J Clin Nutr October 2003 78: 4 728-733
Kelly L Johnston, et al

[20] Caffeine Ingestion Before an Oral Glucose Tolerance Test Impairs Blood Glucose Management in Men with Type 2 Diabetes
J. Nutr. 134:2528-2533, October 2004
Lindsay E. Robinson, et al

[21] Caffeine Impairs Glucose Metabolism in Type 2 Diabetes
Diabetes Care August 2004 vol. 27 no. 8 2047-2048
James D. Lane

[22] Coconuts, and diet on Polynesian atolls: a natural experiment: the Pukapuka and Tokelau Island studies
American Journal of Clinical Nutrition, 1981;34:1552-1561.
Prior IA, et al.

[23] Coconut oil consumption and coronary heart disease
Philippine Journal of Internal Medicine, 1992;30:165-171.
Kaunitz H, Dayrit CS

[24] Concerning the Possibility of a Nut...
Arch Intern Med. 1992;152(7):1371-1372.
William P. Castelli, MD

[25] Saturated fat, carbohydrates and cardiovascular disease.
Neth J Med. 2011 Sep; 69(9):372-8.
Kuipers RS, et al.

[26] Role of dietary fatty acids and acute hyperglycemia in modulating cardiac cell death.
Nutrition. 2004 Oct; 20(10):916-23.
Ghosh S et al.

[27] Reduction of myocardial necrosis in male albino rats by manipulation of dietary fatty acid levels. Lipids. 1982 May;17(5):372-82.
Kramer JK, et al.

[28] Diet and disease--the Israeli paradox: possible dangers of a high omega-6 polyunsaturated fatty acid diet.
Isr J Med Sci. 1996 Nov; 32(11):1134-43.
Yam D, Eliraz A, Berry EM.

[29] A Systematic Review of the Evidence Supporting a Causal Link between Dietary Factors and Coronary Heart Disease.
Arch Intern Med. 2009; 169(7):659-669.
Mente A, et al.

[30] Meta-analysis of prospective cohort studies evaluating the association of saturated fat with cardiovascular disease
Am J Clin Nutr 13 January 2010
Siri-Tarino PW, et al.

[31] http://www.framinghamheartstudy.org/about/index.html

[32] Choice of cooking oils--myths and realities.
J Indian Med Assoc. 1998 Oct; 96(10):304-7.
Sircar S, Kansra U.

[33] Cholesterol, coconuts, and diet on Polynesian atolls: a natural experiment: the Pukapuka and Tokelau island studies.
American Journal of Clinical Nutrition. 1981 Aug; 34(8):1552-61.
Prior IA, Davidson F, et al.

[34] Nicotine and Type 2 Diabetes
Toxicol. Sci. (2008) 103 (2): 225-227
Joseph L. Borowitz1 and Gary E. Isom

[35] Scientific Opinion on the substantiation of health claims related to beta glucans and maintenance of normal blood cholesterol concentrations and maintenance or achievement of a normal body weight
EFSA Journal 2009; 7(9):1254 [18 pp.]. doi:10.2903/j.efsa.2009.1254
Jean-Louis Bresson

[36] Acute cholesterol responses to mental stress and change in posture.
Arch Intern Med. 1992 Apr; 152(4):775-80.
Muldoon MF, et al.

[37] Lifetime exposure to traumatic psychological stress is associated with elevatedInflammation in the Heart and Soul Study
Brain, Behaviour, and Immunity 26 (2012) 642–649
Aoife O'Donovan, et al.

[38] A Paleolithic diet confers higher insulin sensitivity, lower C-reactive protein and lower blood pressure than a cereal-based diet in domestic pigs Nutr Metab (Lond). 2006; 3: 39. doi: 10.1186/1743-7075-3-39 Tommy Jönsson, et al.

[39] Effect of Periodontal Treatment on Glycemic Control of Diabetic Patients: A
systematic review and meta-analysis.
Diabetes Care February 2010 vol. 33 no. 2 421-427.
Wijnand J. Teeuw et al

[40] Slow-wave sleep and the risk of type 2 diabetes in humans
PNAS January 22, 2008 vol. 105 no. 3 1044-1049
Esra Tasali, et al

[41] Effects of Intensive Glucose Lowering in Type 2 Diabetes
N Engl J Med 2008; 358:2545-59.
Stewart, et al.

[42] Surgery as an Effective Early Intervention for Diabesity: Why the reluctance?
Diabetes Care February 2005 28,
John B. Dixon

[43] A low-carbohydrate, ketogenic diet to treat type 2 diabetes
Nutr Metab (Lond). 2005; 2: 34. doi: 10.1186/1743-7075-2-34
Mary C Vernon, et al.

[44] A low-carbohydrate, ketogenic diet to treat type 2 diabetes
Nutr Metab (Lond). 2005; 2: 34 December 1. doi: 10.1186/1743-7075-2-34
William S Yancy, Jr, et al.

[45] Reversal of Diabetic Nephropathy by a Ketogenic Diet
PLoS ONE 6(4): e18604. doi:10.1371/journal.pone.0018604
Charles V. Mobbs, et al.

[46] Reversal of type 2 diabetes: normalisation of beta cell function in association
with decreased pancreas and liver triacylglycerol
Diabetologia DOI 10.1007/s00125-011-2204-7
E. L. Lim , R. Taylor et al

[47] The effect on health of alternate day calorie restriction: eating less and more
than needed on   alternate days prolongs life.
Med Hypotheses. 2006;67(2):209-11. Epub 2006 Mar 10.
Johnson JB, et al

[48] A Low-Glycemic Load Diet Reduces Serum C-Reactive Protein and Modestly
Increases Adiponectin in Overweight and Obese Adults
J. Nutr. 2012 142: 2 369-374; first published online December 21, 2011.
doi:10.3945/jn.111.149807
Johanna W. Lampe, et al.

[49] Epigallocatechin gallate supplementation alleviates diabetes in rodents.
J Nutr. 2006 Oct;136(10):2512-8.
Wolfram S, et al.

[50] Elevated intakes of supplemental chromium improve glucose and insulin variables in individuals with type 2 diabetes.
Diabetes November 1997 46:1786-1791; doi:10.2337/diabetes.46.11.1786
R A Anderson, et al.

[51] Chromium, glucose intolerance and diabetes
J Amer Coll Nutr. 1998;17:548-555
Anderson RA

[52] Chromium in the prevention and control of diabetes
Diabetes and Metabolism. 2000;26(1)22-27
Anderson RA.

[53] Effect of treatment with 3-hydroxy-3-methylglutaryl coenzyme A reductase inhibitors on serum coenzyme Q10 in diabetic patients.
Arzneimittelforschung. 1999 Apr;49(4):324-9.
Miyake Y, et al

[54] Resveratrol Improves Mitochondrial Function and Protects against Metabolic Disease by Activating SIRT1 and PGC-1α p1109
Cell, 15 December, 2006 Volume 127, Issue 6
Marie Lagouge, et al

[55] Vanadyl sulfate improves hepatic and muscle insulin sensitivity in type 2 diabetes
J Clin Endocrinol Metab. 2001 Mar; 86(3):1410-7.
Cusi K, et al.

[56] Vinpocetine inhibits NF-κB–dependent inflammation via an IKK-dependent but PDE- independent mechanism
PNAS 2010 107 (21) 9795-9800; doi:10.1073/pnas.0914414107
Kye-Im Jeon, et al

[57] Fractionation and Purification of the Polysaccharides with Marked Antitumor Activity, Especially Lentinan, from *Lentinus edodes*
Cancer Res November 1970 *30;* 2776
Goro Chihara, et al.

[58] Lentinan prolonged survival in patients with gastric cancer receiving S-1-based   chemotherapy
World Journal of Clinical Oncology (2011), 2(10):339-343.
Ina K, et al.

[59] Hypocholesterolemic action of eritadenine is mediated by a modification of hepatic phospholipid metabolism in rats.
J Nutr. 1995 Aug;125(8):2134-44.
Sugiyama K, et al

[60] Enhancement of muscle mitochondrial oxidative capacity and alterations in insulin action are lipid species-dependent: Potent tissue-specific effects of me dium chain fatty acids
Diabetes August 31, 2009, doi: 10.2337/db09-0784
Nigel Turner, Ji_Ming Ye, et al.

[61] The effect of capsaicin on blood glucose, plasma insulin levels and insulin binding in dog models
Phytotherapy Research Volume 15, Issue 5, pages 391–394, August 2001
I.Tolan, et al.

[62] Mediterranean diet, cocoa and cardiovascular disease: a sweeter life, a longer life, or both?
Journal of Hypertension. 21(12):2231-2234, December 2003.
Ferri, Claudio; Grassi, Guido

[63] Aging and vascular responses to flavanol-rich cocoa
Journal of Hypertension. 24(8):1575-1580, August 2006
Fisher, Naomi DL; Hollenberg, Norman K

[64] Short-term administration of dark chocolate is followed by a significant increase in insulin sensitivity and a decrease in blood pressure in healthy persons
Am J Clin Nutr 2005 81: 611-614,
Davide Grassi, et al

[65] Low-salt diet increases insulin resistance in healthy subjects.
Metabolism. 2011 Jul; 60(7):965-8. doi: 10.1016/j.metabol.2010.09.005.
Epub   2010, Oct 30.
Garg R, et al

[66] Dietary salt intake and mortality in patients with type 2 diabetes.
Diabetes Care. 2011 Mar; 34(3):703-9. doi: 10.2337/dc10-1723.
Epub 2011, Feb 2.
Ekinci EI, et al.

[67] Effects of low-sodium diet vs. high-sodium diet on blood pressure, renin, aldosterone, catecholamines, cholesterol, and triglyceride (Cochrane Review). Am J Hypertens. 2012 Jan;25(1):1-15. doi: 10.1038/ajh.2011.210.
Epub 2011 Nov 9.
Graudal NA, et al

[68] Enhanced Vasodilator Activity of Nitrite in Hypertension HYPERTENSIONAHA.111.00933 Published online before print April 15, 2013, doi: 10.1161/HYPERTENSIONAHA.111.00933
Suborno M. Ghosh, et al.

www.ingramcontent.com/pod-product-compliance
Lightning Source LLC
Chambersburg PA
CBHW032038050726
47590CB00001B/51